TEACH YOURSELF BOOKS

# *Yoga*

D0367802

NTC *NTC Publishing Group*

TEACH YOURSELF BOOKS

# Yoga

## James Hewitt

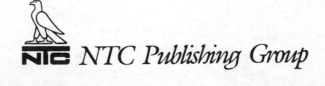 NTC Publishing Group

Long-renowned as the authoritative source for self-guided
learning – with more than 30 million copies sold worldwide –
the *Teach Yourself* series includes over 200 titles in the fields
of languages, crafts, hobbies, sports, and other leisure activities.

This edition was first published in 1993 by NTC Publishing Group,
4255 West Touhy Avenue, Lincolnwood (Chicago), Illinois 60646 –
1975 U.S.A. Originally published by Hodder and Stoughton Ltd.

Library of Congress Catalog Number: 92–82522


Printed and bound in Great Britain
by Cox & Wyman Ltd, Reading, Berkshire

# CONTENTS

# Acknowledgments

I thank the following for giving permission to quote extracts:

Mr Alain Danielou and Christopher Johnson Publishers Ltd, from *Yoga: The Method of Re-integration*; Dr W. Y. Evans-Wentz and Oxford University Press, from *The Tibetan Book of The Dead*; Dr Lily Abegg and Thames and Hudson Ltd, from *The Mind of East Asia*; Mr Mouni Sadhu and George Allen & Unwin Ltd, from *In Days of Great Peace*; Dr Innes H. Pearse and Lucy H. Crocker, B.Sc. and George Allen & Unwin Ltd, from *The Peckham Experiment*; Mr Romain Rolland and Cassell and Co. Ltd., from *Prophets of the New India*; Mr Romain Rolland and George G. Harrap and Co. Ltd, from *Jean-Christophe*; the late Dr Alexis Carrel and Hamish Hamilton Ltd, from *Man The Unknown*; the late Dr Maurice Nicoll and Vincent Stuart, Publishers Ltd, from *Living Time and the Integration of the Life*; the late Mr Aldous Huxley and Chatto and Windus Ltd, from *Ends and Means*; Mr George A. Dorsey and Harper and Brothers, New York, from *Why We Behave Like Humans*; Ms Nancy Phelan and Mr Michael Volin and Stanley Paul Ltd, from *Yoga for Women*; Mr Katsuki Sekida and John Weatherhill Inc., from *Zen Training*; Maharishi Mahesh Yogi and Penguin Books Ltd, from *On the Bhagavad Gita*; Mr I. K. Taimini and the Theosophical Publishing House, from *The Science of Yoga*; Dr Herbert Benson and William Morrow Inc., from *The Relaxation Response*: the late Sri Aurobindo and the Sri Aurobindo Ashram, Pondicherry, India as well as Advaita Ashrama, Calcutta for extracts from Swami Vivekananda's *Raja Yoga*.

# —— INTRODUCTION ——

In Europe and America since the 1950s there has been a remarkable growth of interest in the practice of Yoga, a system of bodily, mental, and spiritual training whose origins are lost in remotest Indian history. Most of the interest and practice centres on the postures and breathing exercises of Hatha Yoga, one of several traditional schools. After only a short period of regular practice, health and vitality improve, suppleness increases, muscles firm and tone, and there is a feeling of lightness, relaxation, and poise that suffuses consciousness as well as the body. The value of Yoga meditation has been more slowly appreciated in the West, but interest and practice in this aspect of Yoga is now growing fast.

Yoga has proved itself to be no here-today-gone-tomorrow fad. Several million Europeans and Americans have derived great physical, mental, and spiritual benefits from its simpler methods. The fact is that Yoga *works* – and good news spreads fast. Most people take up Yoga because they have heard its praises sung by friends and acquaintances.

*Teach Yourself Yoga* concentrates both on the postures, breath controls, and other practices for health and bodily mastery that belong to the school of Hatha Yoga and on the successive stages of sense withdrawal, concentration, meditation, and absorption of Raja Yoga, which produce mental mastery and poise. Traditionally, the exercises of Hatha Yoga act as a purification and preparation for the meditation of Raja Yoga, the 'Royal Way', though they may also be practised for the benefits described above.

There are other Yogas or 'ways', each with their individual methods. Descriptions of many of these techniques are included in *Teach Yourself Meditation*, a companion volume to *Teach Yourself Yoga*. In *Teach Yourself Meditation* are described the essential conditions for undertaking meditation in order to induce states of deep relaxation and pure awareness, together with a range of techniques from which readers may choose by experiment those most suitable to their needs.

The combination of self-discipline, posture, breath control, and meditation is a mainstream tradition in Indian Yoga, and received its classic systematisation in the *Yoga Sutras* written by Patanjali about two to three hundred years BC. We have used Patanjali's famous 'eight limbs' of Yoga as the scaffolding for the construction of this book. The classic tradition provides the roots and foundation for practice, though we should bear in mind that the old textbooks were written for people living many centuries ago in a style far removed from that of the modern technological age. It is hoped that *Teach Yourself Yoga* will be found useful by readers who will welcome both a grounding in basic practice and at the same time the opportunity to learn exactly what Yoga – in its purest form and as practised in its Indian homeland – is about. I hope the reader will learn this from the book even if he or she does not feel particularly inclined to study the mystical elements of metaphysics and philosophy that have been Yoga's *raison d'être* for thousands of years. Many of the popular textbooks on Yoga that have appeared in the West present Yoga as a keep-fit system and describe sketchily and inadequately, if at all, Yoga's mystical dimensions.

However, the main emphasis in *Teach Yourself Yoga* will be on *practice*. This is as it should be within Yogic tradition. 'Practice alone is the means of success,' says the *Hatha Yoga Pradipika*, a key text of its school. And the mystical philosophy of Yoga and of Eastern religion in general is based not on arid theorising but on *experiencing* certain states of consciousness which are revealed by means of meditative practice.

Newcomers to Yoga are advised to lose little time in starting the postures, the relaxation, and the breathing exercises, whose effects in releasing stress and in promoting psycho-physiological poise and well-being are soon experienced. Once these exercises have been mastered, the practice of meditation may then be introduced and the philosophical ideas that give Yoga its traditional motivation may then be studied unhurriedly.

A summary of the contents of each chapter may prove helpful to readers:

**Chapter 1** describes what Yoga is and what it is not. Yoga is both a practice and a goal: the word means 'union'. This is Yoga's mystical dimension, which predominates in India, but not in the West where Yoga is practised more for health, relaxation, emotional stability, and psychological poise. Though the word Yoga may be construed as referring to the union of body and mind in harmonious health and efficiency, at its highest level it refers to the unitary consciousness of the mystic, Hindu or otherwise, in which the ego is transcended and one's essential spiritual nature is realised. This 'union', which has been the goal of Yoga for thousands of years, is realised when body and mind become perfectly quiescent, though the meditator is conscious and alert. The techniques of Yoga, whether postures, breath controls, or meditation, have this aim of great inner stillness.

In Chapter 1, too, the main Yoga paths are described; each path is suited to a different temperament, though there may be some overlapping of paths. Some famous Yoga masters – especially Swami Vivekananda in the nineteenth century and Sri Aurobindo in the twentieth century – have taught a synthesis of various Yogas. Most of the Yogas are described in the *Bhagavad Gita*, a work which calls itself 'a Yoga scripture'. The first four of the six Yogas or paths to union listed in Chapter 1 are given further attention in my companion volume, *Teach Yourself Meditation*. These Yogas are: Jnana, union by knowledge of one's essential nature; Bhakti, union by spiritual devotion; Karma, union by action and service; and Mantra, union by sound. But numbers five and six, which are Hatha or union by bodily mastery and Raja or union by mental mastery, are the subjects of the present book and the sources of its exercises. These exercises, by drawing on our natural psycho-physiological resources, offer the most effective way of coping with stress, which has become a major killer in civilised societies.

**Chapter 2** gives the eight limbs of Yoga, the eightfold path laid down by Patanjali, the 'Father of Yoga', in his classic systematisation of Yoga teaching and practice in that mainstream tradition with which *Teach*

*Yourself Yoga* is concerned. The third and fourth limbs are, respectively, the well-known postures and breath controls. Limbs five to eight are progressive stages in allowing the mind to become quiet and so uncover pure consciousness, known as Samadhi which is the highest stage. The first two limbs are ethical disciplines, moral guidelines for the serious student and the self-discipline that the practice of Yoga requires. But there is no browbeating concerning this 'morality' – Patanjali is describing how a 'realised' or 'perfected' Yogi will live. And Yoga masters rely on the capacity of Yoga practice to change life-styles.

Patanjali's 'eightfold path' has for many centuries provided the framework for the mainstream tradition of Yoga practice in India, and it provides a useful scaffolding for constructing this book.

**Chapter 3** describes the nature of Hatha Yoga, the school of practice whose main components are the postures and breathing exercises. Diet and personal hygiene are also the concern of this form of Yoga. The exercises of Hatha Yoga are so helpful in promoting health and physical fitness and in inducing relaxation of body and mind that for some people they represent all that is important in Yoga. A majority of practitioners in the West and a few in the East have this view of Hatha Yoga.

The exercises of Hatha Yoga bring body and mind into harmony. A key principle in energising the body through the disciplines of Hatha Yoga is that of a prana or cosmic energy. Hatha Yoga promotes the harmonious health of the spine, the nervous system, and the endocrine glands, whose efficient functioning has an important bearing on vitality, health, and longevity. The regular practice of the postures wards off stiffness in the muscles and the joints and slows down the ageing process. The postures and breathing exercises are also conducive to peace of mind, whilst the practices of Hatha Yoga lead naturally to those of Raja Yoga (Royal Yoga), covered by Patanjali's limbs five to eight, which calms the mind through the techniques of meditative awareness.

In **Chapter 4** a range of postures (asanas) are described and illustrated. They include such well-known basic poses as the Shoulderstand, the Plough, the Headstand, the Tree, and the Triangle. Standard performance is described, and in some cases both simplified and slightly more advanced versions are shown. There is also a section describing those postures that require more suppleness than those of the standard programme. A summary of the beneficial effects of each posture follows its description. The chapter concludes with a guide to the therapeutic powers claimed for the postures.

Much of the benefit derived from posturing depends on the manner in which the postures are performed. Forcing may cause aches and strains. Be content to make progress gradually. Whatever stage of suppleness you have reached, perform the postures to the comfortable limit of your capacity and you will benefit greatly. You will soon experience the rewards of improved health, relaxation, and suppleness that have made Yoga posturing so popular; and soon you will also experience the calming and integrating influence that Yoga exercises over your state of mind.

Work your way through the postures and discover those which come most easily to you. To attempt those that you find difficult may still prove valuable if you do not force yourself. The planning of programmes for daily use and further points about performance will be found in Chapter 8.

**Chapter 5** is devoted entirely to relaxation, one of the most valuable skills that modern man can acquire if he is to withstand stress. All the exercises and practices of Yoga promote relaxation and poise, but with the prevalence nowadays of tension and its symptoms of high blood pressure, headaches, and so on, I felt that a separate chapter should be given to the Relaxation Posture (Savasana). This posture should be practised for a few minutes at the conclusion of any session of posturing and at any time when there is a need to 'let go'. Savasana is the neuromuscular skill of letting go from tension, flooding body and mind with feelings of peace. Awareness travels over nineteen body parts from scalp to toes and then in reverse order from toes to scalp, and this is accompanied by a release from tension in each part.

**Chapter 6** deals with Yoga Breathing (Pranayama). The breath controls are often neglected by persons concentrating on the eye-catching postures, but Hatha Yoga derives its name from the former and they should be given an importance at least equal with the postures. *Ha* means 'sun' and *tha* means 'moon', symbolising the positive and negative energies respectively, which are controlled and balanced in Pranayama. Pranayama is 'the control of prana', the vital principle in the universe. It is also the art of breathing correctly, an art which many people who breathe shallowly need to learn if they are to enjoy full alertness and vitality.

The description of the sitting postures of Yoga is reserved for this chapter, as they keep the body steady and compact for the practice of the breath controls, just as they do for the practice of meditation. The cross-legged postures come easily to the Oriental, who is used to sitting on the ground from childhood. Most Westerners can manage the Easy Posture and are able to move on to more advanced sitting postures by gradually accustoming their limbs to the cross-legged position. These postures are valuable exercises in themselves, contributing to the flexibility of the hip joints and to the health of the pelvic region. Persons feeling discomfort in sitting cross-legged may use a straight-backed chair. The most important thing in Yogic sitting is to keep the back upright and straight.

**Chapter 7** gives an account of what Hatha Yoga has to say about personal cleanliness and diet. Performance of some of the cleansing duties (shat karmas) in the traditional way are only of academic interest to most Westerners, though modern adaptation is possible in some cases. It should be remembered that these cleansing practices were devised many centuries ago for Yogis studying and practising in forest ashrams under conditions very different from those prevailing today; but their extraordinary thoroughness suppresses any tendency to superiority about personal hygiene which we might feel today. Few Westerners are prepared to swallow long strips of surgical gauze or to take water into the colon by muscle control, though such traditional methods are still used at some schools of Yoga in India.

The muscle controls of Abdominal Retraction and Isolation of the Recti are also described in Chapter 7, as they have a link with one of the cleansing duties. These abdominal controls are among the most valuable discoveries of Yoga – no exercises work more directly in cultivating the health and vigour of the abdominal region. They eliminate constipation and indigestion, reduce surplus fat, and enhance sexual fitness.

Chapter 7 concludes with a summary of the principles of Yogic diet and eating habits. As with the moral precepts, Yoga relies more on the general practice of Yoga to influence the choice of foods rather than on specific commands to eat this or eat that. Yoga is free from faddism, and moderation is the rule in diet as in other aspects of living.

By the time the reader reaches **Chapter 8** he or she should have tried out the basic exercises and feel himself or herself to be a practitioner of Yoga. Chapter 8 provides guidance on how to make the most of the exercises. It shows how to plan basic programmes of fifteen minutes or twenty minutes, based on the postures described in Chapter 4. For occasions when time is limited on any day, a programme may be followed lasting ten minutes. There is even a rapid vitalising programme lasting only five minutes, in which body stretching and a breathing exercise are combined. The daily programme may be extended to thirty minutes by introducing some of the more advanced postures. The best sequence in the breathing exercises is indicated, as well as advice on mastering the sitting postures and the abdominal controls of Retraction and Isolation of the Recti. This chapter also introduces the Cat Stretch, which combines several postures and is useful when time for practice is limited.

**Chapter 9** introduces Raja Yoga, the 'Royal Way'. The disciplines of Hatha Yoga prepare and purify the body for the meditation of Raja Yoga. The unrest of the mind becomes obvious to anyone who sits quietly and observes its activity. Other discoveries are that there is not one 'I' but many at work and that the mind is more mechanical than is usually realised. The concept of levels of consciousness, familiar in the East but unfamiliar in the West, is introduced. The differing social attitudes of East and West, introvert and extravert respectively, are also discussed. Meditation, for example, is accepted as a healthful and spiritually valuable practice in the East. Chapter 9 ends with an assurance that Raja Yoga is based on the firm foundation of reason and that its fundamental truths arise out of experience.

**Chapter 10** describes the right conditions for the practice of meditation, how much time to give to it, the best place to do it, and how to both sit and breathe for best results. Sense-withdrawal, Patanjali's fifth limb of Yoga, is then described. It is the initial stage of turning inwards and shutting down on the external bombardment from sense impressions. An important technique of Yoga meditation is then described in which the stream of thoughts is observed in passive awareness. After a time the number of thoughts decreases without any deliberate control on the meditator's part; then gaps of tranquillity and silence open between thoughts. The exercise indicates the existence of Self beyond the ego, the realisation of which is the goal of Yoga.

In **Chapter 11** is described *Dharana*, the key meditative practice of concentration. This is the sixth of the eight limbs of Yoga. The flow of attention is directed on to one object or idea and rests there. When attention dwells effortlessly on the object of meditation for some time the stage of *Dhyana* is reached, which may be translated as contemplation or meditation. This is the gateway to the final stage of Samadhi or Realisation.

The technique of gazing on an object, such as an apple, is described, as are various techniques of inner gazing or visualisation, in which the eyes are closed. Listening to sounds, external and internal, is another method of concentrative meditation described in this chapter; the technique of repeating mantras, which are words and phrases, is also discussed. Silent repetition of a word is the basis of the method of Transcendental Meditation, which has many adherents in the West. TM, as it is known, is then studied, and also the use of biofeedback equipment for auto-control of brain wave patterns, changing them to those recorded in meditating Yogins.

Before going on to the eighth limb of Patanjali's 'eightfold path', **Chapter 12** looks at the psychic powers which are said to result from the application of concentration, contemplation, and absorption on selected objects. This is called Samyama, which may be translated as 'mind-poise'. The reasons why Yoga meditation is favourable to extra-sensory perception are explained, and why scientific research into ESP supports Yoga's claims. There follows a concise account of Kundalini Yoga, an occult Yoga based on the awakening of energy in chakras (literally 'wheels') of psychic power in the subtle or astral body.

**Chapter 13** brings us to Samadhi, the eighth of the eight limbs of Yoga, which may be translated as Self-realisation or Absorption. This is the peak of Yoga meditation. It has its own stages of 'with seed' and 'without seed', which are explained. The ego-self is transcended and yet the outcome is not unconsciousness but pure consciousness without thought, word, or image. It is a form of knowledge in which we experience our true selves. The experience is often described as living in the eternal now. Descriptions of Samadhi accord with the experiences of unitary consciousness found in other mystical traditions, whether of East or West. We give here the Hindu Vedanta expression of it, quoting the *Upanishads*, which many people consider to be the purest expression of the 'perennial philosophy' of mysticism.

**Chapter 14**, the concluding chapter, discusses the effect that repeated experience of Samadhi in meditation has on everyday living.

The glossary that follows provides succinct definitions of the Sanskrit Yoga terms used in the text.

# 1

## —— WHAT IS YOGA? ——

### ————— Self-realisation —————

Yoga is firmly incorporated in Indian religion, folklore and vernacular literature. A French scholar, Professor Masson-Ourel, has described Yoga as 'the permanent basis of Indian culture'. Certainly, the different forms of Yoga have played a major part in forming the spirit of modern India.

The origins of this 'life science', as Yoga is often called, are lost in remotest antiquity. Excavations in the Indus basin, made in the twentieth century, uncovered intact ceramics about five thousand years old on which are depicted some of the postures of Yoga. But it is only in recent years that Europeans and Americans in great numbers have discovered the value of practising certain forms of Yoga. They have not, with a few exceptions, become authentic Yogins in the strictest sense, but they practise regularly some of the physical and psychical exercises of some schools of Yoga. Most Indian Yogis devotedly follow a spiritual path and discipline, while many Westerners practising Yoga have much in mind the benefits in health and psycho-physiological relaxation and poise.

The benefits discovered by Westerners taking up Yoga are not unknown to Indians – Hindu scriptures dating back thousands of years describe them; however, they are looked upon as secondary to Yoga's spiritual and mystical goals. In the *Upanishads*, which date from about 800–500 BC, there are many references to the practices of Yoga. In the *Svetasvatara Upanishad*, for example, a distinction is made between 'first results' and the supreme goal of mystical union in Yoga:

> The first results of Yoga they call lightness, healthiness, steadiness, a good complexion, an easy pronunciation, a sweet odour, and slight excretions.

> As a metal disk (mirror), tarnished by dust, shines bright again after it has been cleaned, so is the one incarnate person satisfied and free from grief, after he has seen the real nature of the self.

> And when by means of the real nature of his self he sees, as by a lamp, the real nature of Brahman, then having known the unborn, eternal god, who is beyond all natures, he is freed from all fetters.

This ancient text shows clearly that the Yogis of old were well aware of the improvement in physical and mental health – experienced as lightness, relaxation, and poise – that the practice of Yoga induces; these are benefits that come almost immediately ('first results'). But such changes are secondary to the supreme goal of spiritual freedom and mystical union between individual spirit (Atman) and universal spirit (Brahman).

For the Hindu mystic the supreme goal of living is absorption in Brahman, the all-pervading ground of being. The Sanskrit and Yogic term for this absorption is Samadhi. In it there ends the duality between subject and object, and between perceiver and perceived that exists in ordinary consciousness. The *Upanishads*, together with other Yoga scriptures and textbooks make it clear that the experience called Samadhi is that of a fourth state of consciousness (Turiyavastha), transcending the three states of waking, dreaming, and sleeping without dreams. Of this fourth state of consciousness the *Mandukya Upanishad* says: 'It is One without a second. It is the Self. Know it alone!'

This is the One, mentioned by all forms of mysticism, which goes by various names according to religion and culture. The experience of unitary consciousness has been reported in every age and from most parts of the world. However differently the experience is portrayed by the various religions, the fundamental features of the experience itself are shared by the mystics; the most central feature is knowledge of *union*.

Yoga is a system of psycho-physiological training that has as its goal the uncovering of mystical consciousness. The word 'Yoga' means 'union' or 'identification', and is derived from the same Indo-European root as the English verb 'to yoke'. The union of the individual soul (Atman) and the universal soul (Brahman) is a blissful and ineffable experience. Atman is usually translated as meaning Self, but does not refer to the conditioned ego, which is transcended. The goal of Yoga in its full mystical dimension is therefore Self-realisation (Samadhi). And, as the *Upanishads* state again and again and again, Atman and Brahman, Self and Overself, are all one. When the body and the mind become perfectly quiet, the Yogi discovers the answer to the question 'Who (or what) am I?'; the essence of existence lies in the substratum of being. The training for making body and mind perfectly quiet is called Yoga.

As Yoga's supreme goal of mystical consciousness is shared by persons who are Hindus, Buddhists, Taoists, Jews, Christians, and Sufists, there may be said to be Yogas within each of these traditions, though Indian Hindu Yoga is the main source of the practices described in this book. The methods of meditation used in these other Yogas are described in my companion volume *Teach Yourself Meditation*. The techniques of Indian Hindu Yoga are incorporated to varying degrees in the spiritual training of Buddhism, which originated in India, in Taosim, in Zen, in Judaism, in Sufism, in the mystical wing of Islam, and in Christianity (particularly the Orthodox Church).

Descriptions of Yoga methods are to be found in the sacred works of the Hindu, such as the *Vedas*, the *Upanishads*, the *Bhagavad Gita*, and the *Tantras*. 'From the point of view of their ultimate significance all the Hindu scriptures, indeed, the scriptures of all religions, may be said to be treatises of Yoga,' writes Alain Danielou in his *Yoga: The Method of Re-Integration*. 'The aim of all religions is to bring man towards union with, or re-integration into, the Supreme Being. Religious practices or moral disciplines are only preliminary stages in this process.'

There is nothing in Yoga that should offend people of the Christian or any other faith. Yoga teaches the unity of all life and sets out a programme of practical exercises whereby you can experience this. Anyone can benefit from Yoga. The believer who practises it will be brought closer to God.

Ramakrishna says: 'Through Yoga a Hindu becomes a better Hindu, a Christian a better Christian, a Mohammedan a better Mohammedan, and a Jew a better Jew.'

Equally, an agnostic or atheist may practise Yoga and derive great benefit. This may seem strange until you come to understand just what the Yoga techniques involve. The system of physical mastery known as Hatha Yoga and the system of psychical mastery known as Raja Yoga – the two Yogas with which this work is chiefly concerned – constitute in themselves, regardless of the mystical goal for which they were originally created, efficacious ways to health, relaxation, mental power and peace of mind. An atheist may even seek Samadhi, but will look on it as a means of refreshment and renewal, as a mental state in which there is a strong and blissful feeling of 'oneness' with the universe, or perhaps as a brief contact with a higher state of consciousness towards which man is evolving.

Whatever your belief, whatever your sex, age or race, put Yoga into practice and it will lead to a more abundant living.

# ───── The Yoga paths ─────

While mystical union is the goal of Yoga, there are many paths to its attainment.

Here are the six main paths:

| | |
|---|---|
| Jnana Yoga | union by knowledge |
| Bhakti Yoga | union by devotion |
| Karma Yoga | union by action |
| Mantra Yoga | union by sound |
| Hatha Yoga | union by bodily control |
| Raja Yoga | union by mental control |

From this you will see that the ancient Yogis in their wisdom devised many paths for the many different temperaments of men.

*Jnana* is obviously for the intellectual. The truths of existence and the nature of the Self are examined. The student must see for himself that he is not the body, feeling, personality, or intellect, but their user. The pure

Self beyond the ego is concealed like the sun behind cloud. Only by the most diligent self-training can it be revealed and experienced as reality.

*Bhakti* involves faith and worship. It is the Yoga of devotion, involving concentration and meditation on the Divine. It is as much the way of the emotions as Jnana is of the intellect. It asks for service to your fellow men and unselfishness.

*Karma* is for the active and the extravert. It is work performed for the service of mankind, and at the same time it is worship. The craftsman worships with his tools, the farmer with his plough.

Vivekananda believed in a synthesis of the various Yogas – Jnana, Bhakti, Karma, Raja – to achieve self-realisation, and he warned against life-negation. Meditation should not lead to introspective egoism, but to an annihilation of egoism and the feeling of identification with all people, in whom one recognises one's own Self. Thus the Yogi should seek to serve others. Not 'I', but 'Thou', said Vivekananda, should be the watchword of all well-being.

> Here is the world and it is full of misery. Go out into it as Buddha did and struggle to lessen it or die in the attempt. Forget yourselves; this is the first lesson to be learnt, whether you are a theist or an atheist, whether you are an agnostic or a Vedantist, a Christian or a Mohammedan. (*Practical Vedanta*)

*Mantra* concentrates the mind by means of Japa, the repetition of special words and sentences, prayers and incantations. The Japa may be voiced, whispered, or mental. Mantra deals with the subject of sound vibrations, and there is much in this path that will fascinate the musician.

Maharishi Mahesh Yogi's technique of Transcendental Meditation, which has been taught to more than one million Westerners, is based on mental repetition of a mantra – a word whose repetition takes the meditator, in awareness, to the source of thought, which is pure being.

*Hatha* enables you to understand your body and gain mastery over it.

It is Hatha Yoga which makes the most immediate appeal to the Occidental, and it is this Yoga that is best known in the West. Physical exercises, hygiene and breathing practices are all part of Hatha Yoga. The ancient Yogis had an astounding knowledge of the workings of the human body. It was this knowledge – together with the study of the stretching movements of jungle animals (especially those of the cat family) – that enabled them to formulate the most perfect of all systems for achieving and maintaining bodily health and fitness. The superiority of this system over others lies in the fact that it aims at developing not only muscular strength or size, but the health and efficiency of the internal organs such as the heart, lungs, glands and nerves. Furthermore it does not require any apparatus and can be practised in a confined space.

*Raja* Yoga is closely linked with Hatha Yoga and they are often practised together. Some Yogic authorities lay great stress on the bodily Hatha Yoga, while others of the Raja Yoga school consider only a little Hatha necessary and rely entirely on psychic development. Just as the Hatha aims at mastering the body, so Raja aims at mastering the mind. It seeks to gain control over the stream of thoughts that flow through the human mind. It seeks to check that flow and quiet the mind by means of Concentration (Dharana) and Contemplation (Dhyana). By these practices a state of Super-consciousness (Samadhi) may be achieved.

Just as Everest could not have been conquered by weaklings, so the Yogi knows that to reach his spiritual goal his body must be at its fittest and most efficient so that the mind can be conquered and made the servant of the Self.

Hatha and Raja Yoga are therefore means to an end, but even if you ignore the end and think only of the means, you have on the one hand the world's finest physical-culture system, and on the other hand a method of mental mastery that far surpasses expensive mind-training courses.

Romain Rolland, in *Prophets of the New India*, says: 'Normally we waste our energies. Not only are they squandered in all directions by the tornado of exterior impressions; but even when we manage to shut doors and windows, we find chaos within ourselves, a multitude like the one that greeted Julius Caesar in the Roman Forum; thousands of unexpectedly and mostly "undesirable" guests invade and trouble us. No inner activity can be seriously effective and continuous until we have first reduced our house to order, and then have recalled and reassembled our herd of scattered energies.'

Raja Yoga is designed to do just that – to put our mental house in order and concentrate our scattered energies. It integrates the mind, stills its turbulence, cleanses it, strengthens it. Just as a body that has been cleansed of its toxic waste becomes healthier and stronger, so a mind emptied of its encumbering dross becomes healthier and stronger. Regular Raja Yoga practice builds up a store of mental energy that will remain on tap.

By holding the mind steady in meditative concentration, dormant powers are awakened. Some readers may question this, but Yoga students testify that it is so. Those familiar with the psychology of the sub-conscious will understand the seeming paradox that when the mind is relaxed and held steady in a receptive state many creative and intellec-tual problems will work themselves out to a solution, magically and effortlessly.

*Laya* (Latent) Yoga is a combination of many Yogas – breathing, pos-tures, listening to inner sounds, and so on – including the occult *Kundalini* Yoga. This sets out to awaken what is symbolically described as Kundalini, 'the coiled serpent' said to sleep at the base of the spine, which when aroused travels upwards through the sushumna or spinal channel, passing through various centres or chakras until, when it reaches the centre of consciousness in the brain, a superconscious state is achieved. There is a considerable body of literature on the symbology of the chakras, depicted as a series of many-petalled flowers, bearing numerous symbols. Some modern investigators approximate the chakras with the principal nerve ganglia, others with the glands; but it is probably best to look on the chakras as centres of physical energy within the subtle or astral body. Kundalini Yoga could be dangerous for those who would explore it without the guidance of a highly qualified teacher.

# Health and happiness in an age of stress

The great age of Yoga, ignorance of its true nature and the symbolistic obscurity of much of the writings on the subject give many Westerners – moving as they do in a world of constant unrest – the impression that the system holds nothing for them and is all rather remote, vague and impractical. In this they make a grave mistake, for Yoga is the most practical means of attaining health and happiness in an age of stress.

We should not support those pessimists who believe that civilisation should be destroyed and that we should return to the levels of human development achieved by the cave-man. The harnessing of the forces of nature, such as electricity and atomic energy, to allow us to fly faster than sound and explore space . . . these are wonderful achievements, triumphs for Man in his conquest of the universe. But sometimes he is inclined to forget that he is not a machine, but a living being. In the West millions live at such a hectic pace that they are committing slow suicide. Civilisation imposes pressures and strain unknown to our grandparents. Man can only successfully meet this challenge by paying increasing attention to his physical and mental well-being.

Yoga provides an answer to the problem of stress.

When I first took up daily Yoga practice many years ago, I kept a record of my reactions in a little notebook. Looking at it now, I see the following results.

Almost immediately there was definite increase in vitality; stamina was also greatly increased and I felt quite fresh even at the end of a busy day.

The postures (Asanas) made my muscles firmer and better shaped. I felt (and was) stronger and more supple. My posture became more upright and my physique more athletic.

My weight dropped by ten pounds in three months and my waistline was reduced one inch. The abdominal muscles became firmer and more defined. Bowel elimination became regular. Friends remarked how well I was looking. I felt more buoyant and youthful.

I found that my mind had become more tranquil and my temperament more placid. I was master of my emotions. I rarely gave way to anger, or the other negative emotions. My outlook on life became brighter and I had a greater zest for living. I lived more in the present, less in the past and future. I looked at the world and myself more objectively. My sense of awareness was heightened. Concentration was much improved and I could work more efficiently and for long stretches without experiencing mental fatigue.

I began to feel at one with – and reverent towards – all living things.

I have talked with many people who have taken up regular Yoga practice and the results I achieved are similar to theirs and by no means exceptional. It is because of such benefits as these that scientists, writers, psychologists, artists, musicians, ballet-dancers, singers, sportsmen and sportswomen, indeed people in all walks of life, practise Yoga and greatly praise its help in achieving healthier, happier, and more efficient living.

It is not necessary to live a life of solitude to achieve results from Yoga. You can take an active part in civilised life; the daily practice of Yoga will act as a protection from the numerous stresses of your environment. There has been striking scientific proof of the authenticity of the claim that Yoga-type meditation can act as an effective antidote to stress. Laboratory studies by Dr Herbert Benson at the Harvard Medical School show that Yogic meditation produces what Dr Benson calls the 'Relaxation Response'. In physiological terms the Relaxation Response shows as a marked decrease in the breathing rate and in oxygen consumption (to levels below that in deep sleep), a lowering of the heart rate (on average by about three beats per minute), a decrease in blood pressure in meditators whose levels had been higher than normal, a fall in the level of lactate in the blood (lactate is linked with attacks of anxiety), and the production during meditation of Alpha waves in the brain which are associated with mental relaxation. These distinct physiological changes account for reports by practitioners of Yoga meditation that they soon felt more relaxed and serene and were better able to cope with the pace and stress of living.

Whether you are a businessman, a farmer, a factory worker, a university student or a housewife, Yoga has something to offer. Whatever your age, sex, creed or race, you can achieve the same results by following this wonderful life-science – glowing health, increased energy and stamina, a shapelier body, relaxation, improved concentration and peace of mind.

# 2

# THE EIGHT LIMBS OF YOGA

Patanjali, in his *Yoga Sutras*, which were written between 200 and 300 BC, systematised the teachings and techniques of the tradition that has supplied the exercises which have proved most popular and beneficial in the West in recent times. 'Sutras' may be translated approximately as 'aphorisms'. 'In the basic literature of Yoga, the *Yoga Sutras* of Patanjali stands out as the most authoritative and useful book,' says I. K. Taimini, in *The Science of Yoga* (The Theosophical Publishing House, Wheaton, Illinois). 'In its 196 Sutras the author has condensed the essential philosophy and technique of Yoga in a manner which is a marvel of condensed and scientific exposition.' This condensation, marvel though it is, makes it a very difficult work to read and little headway will be made without the assistance of a commentary, which, fortunately, is provided by most translators. Patanjali intended his work to be a kind of shorthand, to be explained and expanded by Yoga masters orally instructing their pupils.

Patanjali, having in Section 1 of the *Sutras* discussed the goal of Yoga, which is Samadhi, in Section 2 turns to the disciplines that bring it about. These are the eight angas or limbs of Yoga, which provide the framework for mainstream practice. Though called 'the Father of Yoga', Patanjali did not originally conceive it – its origins are lost in remotest antiquity – but he was the first and most important systematiser and codifier.

The eight limbs of Yoga are:

Abstinences (Yamas)
Observances (Niyamas)
Postures (Asanas)
Breath controls (Pranayama)
Sense withdrawal (Pratyahara)
Concentration (Dharana)
Contemplation or Meditation (Dhyana)
Absorption or Self-realisation (Samadhi)

## —————— Ethical disciplines ——————

Each of the limbs of Yoga are in some way a purification. The first two limbs lay down guidance for the moral standards and spiritual conduct expected of the serious student. But nothing rigid or severe is intended: Yoga is free from pressures of sin or guilt, which would be obstacles to progress just as much as a failure to be guided by the abstinences or to follow the observances. And there is a sense in which Patanjali might be said to put the cart before the horse here. For as progress is made in Yoga the quality of the student's ethical life changes, until it reaches full spontaneous flowering in the 'Realised Man'. The whole personality is transformed in the person who has found the Self beyond the ego and realised the identity of Self and Brahman – compassion, gentleness, truthfulness, honesty, purity and other values arise effortlessly. There is no need, therefore, for any reader to feel daunted by the moral guidelines that Patanjali gives as the first two limbs of Yoga. Take note of them and then press on with the practice of the postures, the breath control, and the meditation.

## —— The five abstinences (Yamas) ——

Patanjali lists five Yamas: abstaining from killing, from falsehood, from theft, from incontinence, and from greed.

# Non-violence (Ahimsa)

This means extending compassion to all sentient creatures. It was the favourite precept of Mahatma Gandhi, who said of it: 'Ahimsa is not merely a negative state of harmlessness but it is a positive state of love, of doing good even to the evil-doer.' Patanjali says: 'Near him in whom non-violence has fully taken root, all beings renounce enmity.'

# Truthfulness (Satya)

This means not only speaking truthfully, but has the wider meaning of sincerity in one's dealings with others.

# Non-stealing (Asteya)

This includes but has wider implications than abstinence from theft. It could apply, for example, to refusing undeserved credit.

# Brahmacharya

The fourth of the five abstinences may be given several definitions, according to how narrow or how broad a view you take of it. In a narrow sense it is *chastity* or *continence*. The student joining an ashram or Yoga school is usually expected to transmute sexual energy into spiritual energy; but it would be entirely wrong to identify such an abstinence in any way with a sense of sin about sex. Continence has the meaning of being 'temperate' and leads to broader definitions of brahmacharya as *spiritual conduct, non-sensuality*, and so on. Non-sensuality includes not clinging to sensual pleasures – which means not necessarily avoiding them – and includes the Eastern concepts of non-attachment and non-grasping. A severe opposition to sensuality is a disguised form of attachment and clinging, just as the fanatical 'true believer' is bound to all that he hates. As Brahmacharya may be defined as meaning 'of the character of Brahman' (the 'Brahman' is the Divine Reality), then 'spiritual conduct' serves as a good guide for the fourth Yama.

A few more points are worth making about Yoga's relation to sexuality.

Chastity is not expected of the 'householder Yogi', who continues his normal family duties. Indeed he may use Yoga exercises to heighten sexual fitness and for him the act of sexual intercourse may be used as a form of contemplation of ceremonial power, as it is in Tantrism, one of the major schools of Yoga. An improvement in sexual fitness and fulfilment are among the benefits frequently reported by men and women who have taken to practising Yoga regularly. Yoga promotes the physiological and psychological factors which enhance sexuality; vitality, muscle tone, supple limbs and joints, and efficient functioning of the nervous system, circulation and glands, on the physical side, and freedom from tensions and anxieties and a well-honed awareness, on the psychological side.

Some of the postures described in Chapter 4 are associated with improved sexual fitness: in particular, the Shouderstand, the Plough, the Cobra, the Bow, the Locust, the Spinal Twist, the Thunderbolt and the Supine Thunderbolt. There are also certain bandhas or 'bindings' and mudras or 'seals' which are linked with harnessing sexual energy. I have shown how these muscle controls may be used to promote sexual fitness in *The Complete Yoga Book* (Rider), and a chapter on 'Tantrism: the Yoga of Sex' appears in the same work. Uddiyana Bandha, probably the most important of the bandhas, and its follow-up muscle control of Isolating the Recti, tone the muscles of the pelvic floor and stimulate circulation in that area. They are described in Chapter 4 of this book.

## Non-possessiveness (Aparigrapha)

This is sometimes translated as 'non-hoarding'; it does not mean that the Yogin has no possessions, but just that their importance does not dominate him so that he is their slave.

# — The five observances (Niyamas) —

The five observances are purity, contentment, austerity, study and attentiveness to the Divine.

## Purity (Saucha)

We have already pointed out that all the practices of Yoga aim at purification. The goal is Samadhi, in which pure consciousness is experienced. On a physical level, the hygienic practices of Hatha Yoga include some that do not appear in other cultures and show a remarkable knowledge of human anatomy and functioning. In diet, the Yogi is advised to eat sattvic or pure foods, because they help purify body and soul.

## Contentment (Santosha)

This is one of the hallmarks of the person experienced in Yoga. It is accompanied by simplicity and serenity. The Yogi should be cheerful, uncomplaining, free from strong desires and satisfied with simple needs. Regular practice of Yoga in all its 'limbs' leads to greater harmony within oneself, with others and with the cosmos of which one is an integral part.

## Austerity (Tapas)

This term does not mean self-mortification or excessive asceticism, though it has sometimes been mistaken for such. It refers to simplicity in living and to keeping the will resolutely on the goals of Yoga. 'Self-discipline' is a good definition. In the *Bhagavad Gita*, a work describing the various Yogas, Lord Krishna says of persons who are excessively austere – 'fools they are'. Purification is again implicit, for the Yogin's intent should burn like a steady flame. The word 'tapas' is derived from the root 'tap' meaning to blaze or to shine.

## Study (Svadhyaya)

This includes reading attentively the *Upanishads*, the *Bhagavad Gita*, and other key works of Yoga literature, and also the self-enquiry of 'Who (or What) am I?', in which the skins of the 'ego-onion' are stripped away until essential being (the Self) is exposed to pure awareness.

## *Attentiveness to the Divine (Ishvara Pranidhana)*

This involves surrendering the grip of the ego and trusting in the Self and the divine ground of being.

Limbs three to eight will be discussed at length in the chapters to follow. The postures (Asanas) and the breath controls (Pranayama) belong to the bodily mastery of Hatha Yoga in their highest development, though some Yogins engaging in intensive meditation may restrict these two limbs mainly to the sitting postures of meditation and regulation of the breath so as to quieten the body and the mind. Sense Withdrawal (Pratyahara), Concentration (Dharana), Contemplation (Dhyana), and Self-realisation (Samadhi), sometimes called Identification or Absorption, represent the final stages of Raja Yoga, the 'Royal Way'.

In withdrawing the senses, the Yogi turns his attention inwards. The attention is then held steadily on some object, in concentration that flows effortlessly into the succeeding stage of contemplation or meditation. In Samadhi there is no distinction or separation between the perceiver and that which is perceived. The meditator is taken to the core of consciousness and the ground of being. The experience can be but poorly described in words; it is a kind of knowledge, in which knower and known are one; it is accompanied by deep peace; the Hindu Yogis speak in this context of sat-chit ananda which is awareness or bliss. The body and the senses are quiescent, thought has ceased, and yet there is a bright, lively awareness. The meditator discovers who he is – not ego-self, but Self. The realisation of Self is the eighth and final limb of Yoga.

# 3

# THE PATH TO
## ———— HEALTH ————
# (HATHA YOGA)

Hatha Yoga consists of the six Purification Practices (Shat Karmas), the Postures (Asanas), and the Breath Controls (Pranayama), which bring body and mind into harmony and prepare the latter for the techniques of Raja Yoga (The Royal Path).

The Yoga Sanskrit texts refer to Hatha Yoga as the ladder to Raja Yoga. The *Goraksha Samhita* says:

> The science of Hatha Yoga is the ladder up which those climb who wish to reach the higher regions of the Royal Path (Raja Yoga).

*The Hatha Yoga Pradipika* says:

> Asanas (postures), various kumbhakas (breath controls), and other divine means, all should be utilised in the practice of Hatha Yoga, till the fruit – Raja Yoga – is obtained.

And the *Siva Samhita* says:

> The Hatha Yoga cannot be obtained without the Raja Yoga, nor can the Raja Yoga be attained without the Hatha Yoga.

As already mentioned the word Hatha takes its meaning from the syllables 'ha' (the sun) and 'tha' (the moon); just as Yoga itself means union, Hatha Yoga is a union of sun and moon. This is a symbolic term for the uniting of the positive and negative energies of the body.

Alain Danielou, in his *Yoga: The Method of Re-Integration*, explains:

'The cosmic Principles which, in relation to the earth, manifest themselves in the planetary world as the sun and the moon are found in every aspect of existence. In man, they appear mainly under two forms, one in the subtle body, the other in the gross body. In the subtle body they appear as two channels along which our perceptions channel between the subtle centre at the base of the spinal cord and the centre at the summit of the head. These two channels are called Ida and Pingala. Ida, situated on the left side, corresponds to the cold aspect or the moon and Pingala, on the right side, to the warm aspect or the sun.

'In the gross body, the lunar and solar principles correspond to the respiratory, cool, and the digestive, warm, vital energies, and are called Prana and Apana. It is by co-ordinating these two most powerful vital impulses that the yogi achieves his aim.'

# Harmonious health

I need hardly point out the great value of sound health. Ariphon, the Sicyonian, said: 'Without health, life is not life; life is lifeless,' and Emerson remarked: 'The first wealth is health.'

The Yogis believe that sound health can belong to all men and women. Nature provides an illimitable fund of energy, available to all living things. The fact that man disregards Nature's laws with such recklessness and still manages to exist shows the power of this life force. He may abuse it, mock it, turn his back on it, but it goes on fighting for him. How often have cases been given up as lost by the doctors, only to see life hold on by a tenuous thread and finally triumph.

It is this same life force – the Yogis call it Prana – that brings the tree to bloom, the blossom to fruit, that energises the leaping lamb, that propels the gazelle. Each of us has a share in an ocean of energy.

Vivekananda puts it:

In an ocean there are huge waves, then smaller waves, and still smaller, down to little bubbles; but back of all these is the infinite ocean. The bubble is connected with the infinite ocean at one end, and the huge wave at the other end. So, one may be a gigantic man, and another a little bubble; but each is connected with that infinite ocean of energy which is the common birthright of every animal that exists. Wherever there is life, the storehouse of infinite energy is behind it.

If instead of battling against Nature man invoked her aid his achievements would be infinite.

# – The perfect home exercise system –

Of all home exercise systems Hatha Yoga is the most perfect. It does not require any apparatus, and can be performed in a small space. It does not demand a great expenditure of energy; it therefore suits people of all ages, and is ideal for the exhausting times in which we live.

With its gentle, refreshing nature Hatha Yoga has none of the drawbacks of more strenuous systems, which accumulate fatigue poisons in the muscles. While those who practise the asanas regularly find their bodies becoming shapelier and their muscles firmer and stronger, Hatha Yoga aims primarily at organic health and not mere muscular development. Actually Yoga asanas are postures to be held, and not exercises in the normal meaning of the word. Their stretching action has a relaxing effect, a valuable asset in an age of stress.

Almost all the asanas have a stretching action on the spine, which houses and protects the vital nerve channels. Bodily efficiency depends on each of the billions of cells making up our bodies playing its full part in the community . . . in a word, on harmony. This harmony depends more than anything else on the work of the nervous system. With the brain as the co-ordinating centre, messages pour in by means of billions of nerve fibres. Messages received by the senses are flashed to the brain where they are stored or computed and an immediate answer given. There are cells carrying nourishment, cells busy with the task of removing waste products, cells carrying messages. The nervous system is the telephone service of the cell community. Its telephone network reaches every part of our bodies.

The fine nerves coming from the sense organs group together into cables on the way to the brain exchange, the biggest cable being the spinal cord which is located in and protected by the spinal column. The importance of keeping the spine flexible and in healthy condition is obvious.

One set of nerves – the sensory – make their way with their messages to the brain, and another reaches out with the reply from the brain – the motor nerves. The brain has its own centre for distributing the work. The centre dealing with sight, for example, is to the rear of the cerebrum, the centre for hearing just below the Fissure of Sylvius, and so on.

There is a second nervous system, partly connected with the central nervous system and partly independent. This is the autonomic nervous system. It has nerve centres, called ganglia, located alongside the spinal cord. There are also ganglia in the head, the stomach, and other places. A blow in the region of the stomach ganglia knocks the wind out of you and you are breathless. The autonomic nervous system controls the working of the glands, the heart (the beating of the heart depends on a ganglion located there), and it is also closely connected with the feelings, as manifested in blushing and crying. Some Yogis develop self-mastery to such a degree that they can influence the working of the autonomic nervous system.

Living depends on constant reaction and adjustment to our environment. Without the complex nervous system this would be impossible. The ancient Yogis, in devising their disciplines, gave primary consideration to the maintenance of a healthy and efficient nervous system.

Hatha Yoga promotes the harmonious health of the internal organs and glands, the principal endocrine glands all being acted upon by the various postures.

Of these glands, George A. Dorsey, in his book *Why We Behave Like Human Beings*, says: 'The secretions of the ductless glands are discharged direct into the blood, hence they are also called glands of internal secretion or endocrines (*endon*, within; *krino*, I separate). Endocrine secretions are chemical in nature and are usually called hormones (exciters). They are also called autacoid substances: from *acos*, a remedy – they act like drugs. They are, in fact, drugs, some of them of astounding potency. In fact, no man-made drugs are so powerful as some we make in our own drug-store glands.'

# Rejuvenation

The work of the endocrine glands has a direct bearing on vitality and longevity. Hatha Yoga is the system par excellence of rejuvenation. Daily Yoga exercise not only wards off stiffness of the muscles and joints, one of the troubles of old age, but it also slows down the whole physiological ageing process. Biological and chronological time are two different things, the former varying with each individual. We age at different speeds. One man is a spent force at sixty, while another is comparatively fresh.

In *Man the Unknown*, Alexis Carrel writes: 'Inward time cannot be properly measured in units of solar time. However, it is generally expressed in days and years because these units are convenient and applicable to the classification of terrestrial events. But such a procedure gives no information about the rhythm of the inner processes constituting our intrinsic time. Obviously, chronological age does not correspond to physiological age. Puberty occurs at different epochs in different individuals. It is the same with menopause. True age is an organic and functional state. It has to be measured by the rhythm of the changes of this state. Such rhythm varies according to individuals. Some remain young for many years. On the contrary, the organs of others wear out early in life. The value of physical time in a Norwegian, whose life is long, is far from being identical with that in an Eskimo, whose life is short. To estimate true, or physiological, age, we must discover, either in the tissues or in the humours, a measurable phenomenon, which progresses without interruption during the whole life-time.'

Of equal importance to the benefits to bodily health and efficiency that come from Hatha Yoga practice is the calming and integrating influence on the personality. For Hatha Yoga is a system of bodily purification, leading naturally to Raja Yoga, which is a technique of self-development and conscious evolution.

Tranquillity of mind is of as much importance as bodily care if you wish to live a long and active life. Looking over some cuttings from my files under the heading 'Longevity', I notice a frequently occurring answer to the reporter's inevitable questions to the centenarian: 'To what do you attribute your long life?' The most frequently given reply is 'freedom from worry' . . . in other words, peace of mind.

Worry is a great killer. Dr Kenneth Walker has written that it kills more people than cancer. So, too, does boredom. Old people should have as many interests as possible. Retirement should be taken as an opportunity, not for idleness, but for creative leisure.

Great ages are reached in the Yoga ashrams of the East, where lives of self-mastery and tranquillity are lived, though accurate figures are difficult to obtain. In China, where meditation is an ancient art, the Taoists lived such long lives that the Emperor Ch-Hoang-Ti (who ruled 221–209 BC) thought they must have a secret elixir and sent for it.

The influence of the emotions on health is now well-known to medical science. Emotional stress and conflict can cause not only minor ailments, but serious diseases. Hatha Yoga purifies the body. Raja Yoga purifies the mind and achieves emotional mastery. The renowned Hungarian neuropathist, Dr Francis Volgyesi, once said: 'Yoga is actually the primitive ancestor, thousands of years old, of the brand-new science that we call psycho-therapy.'

To achieve that harmony with nature that is perfect health, the Hatha Yogi in India goes through a rigorous programme. He devotes his life to it, performing many of the exercises for hours daily. This arduous practice gives him a control over body and mind that is extraordinary. (For a fascinating account of what it is like to undergo full training under a guru, or Yoga master, see Theos Bernard's works *Hatha Yoga* and *Heaven Lies Within Us*.)

It is doubtful whether there would be many readers willing to undertake such a programme even if they had the time to spare. However, in Chapter 8 it will be shown how fifteen to thirty minutes daily can be utilised for a Yoga programme of immense benefit to bodily and mental health.

In Chapter 4 are given the best known of the Yoga exercises. Scientific tests have been made with regard to the physiological effects of these exercises and the results show beyond any doubt that they promote health to a wonderful degree.

A few of the postures require considerable strength or suppleness but have been included as they are likely to be of interest to advanced students; and though some of the hygienic practices are unsuited to modern living, they have been described to show what a remarkable understanding of and control over the human body the Yogi possesses.

# 4

# YOGA POSTURES (ASANAS)

Yogic physical exercises – actually they are postures to go into and hold immobile – are unrivalled as a means of improving bodily health and suppleness. Their superiority over other systems – such as calisthenics, weight-training and gymnastics – lies in the fact that they aim at promoting the health and efficiency of the vital internal organs. The postures are performed symmetrically, alternating positions so that both sides of the body receive equal toning. A bend to the left is followed by a bend to the right: a forward bend is followed by a backward bend; a contraction is followed by a stretch, and so on. This prevents lopsided development of the kind produced by tennis, and some other sports. The Yogis who devised these postures displayed a profound knowledge of human anatomy and physiology. In particular, they bore in mind the need for keeping the spine, the nerves and the glands in healthy condition, thus giving organic vigour to the whole body. Moreover, the postures have a calming and integrating influence on the workings of the mind and are traditionally used to prepare the mind for meditation.

Many thousands of men and women, from all walks of life, are now practising the Yoga postures and testify that their practice will rejuvenate the body, reduce obesity, strengthen and tone the muscles, make the spine and the body more supple, tone the nervous system, keep diseases at bay, prevent constipation and dyspepsia, keep the skin glowing and healthy, and promote mental alertness and serenity.

Use common sense when first attempting these postures. If you doubt the suitability of any of them, consult a doctor. Persons suffering from high blood pressure, heart ailments, or diseases of the brain, eyes, and ears should leave out the Headstand.

If you are of normal health and suppleness, you can attempt all the asanas, provided you are careful not to over-strain the body. Be content to progress gradually.

Postures are also often not advised for women during pregnancy. The older books on Yoga warn against exercising during pregnancy, but some of the more recent publications say that *some* of the postures may be continued during pregnancy, as long as common sense is applied and a doctor's consent is received. The exercises, breath controls, and relaxation techniques practised for so-called 'natural childbirth' have close similarities with training in Yoga. However, the following exercises should *not* be practised during pregnancy: Abdominal Retraction and Isolation of the Recti, any postures contracting the abdomen, and any posture that might alter the position of the child, such as the Headstand. On the other hand, the Relaxation Posture is a valuable practice throughout pregnancy, and the cross-legged sitting postures, which loosen the hip joints and stretch and tone the muscles of the pelvic floor, are also helpful. Yogic breathing exercises (pranayama) can be beneficial, though those requiring abdominal contractions should *not* be performed.

Nancy Phelan and Michael Volin, who have had much experience in teaching classes, state in *Yoga for Women* (Stanley Paul): 'If you are a yoga student, wishing to prepare for childbirth but for some reason unable to attend ante-natal classes, you could, with your doctor's approval, achieve almost the same results by concentrating on certain yoga techniques and exercises. These will not of course give you instructions for actual childbirth procedure but will prepare your nerves and muscles in exactly the same way as the ante-natal exercises.

'After the third month it is advisable to give up most of the usual asanas – though some women continue to practise inverted poses, apart from the Headstand, and forward-stretching movements until the sixth or seventh month; but in any case nothing should be done without the doctor's consent, and no exercises attempted that involve strenuous upward stretching, violent stomach contractions or anything that might adversely affect the position of the child. The Headstand is forbidden for this reason.'

There are a number of Yoga postures which require considerable suppleness; some of these are given under the heading of 'Advanced Postures'. When simplified versions of an asana are given, these follow the description of standard performance. Correct performance of even the simplest poses may not be easy for every student, especially for the person who has not led an athletic life or is carrying surplus fat, though some fat beginners do well. Remember that the attempt is doing you good; and if you are inclined to be obese Yoga will soon normalise your figure, as long as you are sensible in matters of diet.

This chapter should be used in conjunction with Chapter 8, which provides advice on making the most of the exercises and gives programmes lasting from five to twenty minutes. The postures on which to draw for programmes are described in the present chapter.

Try out the standard postures – those described up to the advanced postures – in the order given. They include such favourites of Yoga practice as the Tree Posture, the Shoulderstand Posture, the Plough Posture, the Headstand Posture, the Cobra Posture, the Bow Posture, the Back-stretching Posture, and the Standing Forward Bend Posture. You need not perform all of them immediately. Try out from the Tree Posture to the Cobra Posture today and the Bow Posture to the Mountain Posture tomorrow. On subsequent days perform all of them, once only. If you are a beginner, perform the Half Shoulderstand Posture, the Half Headstand Posture, the simplified variation of the Cobra Posture, and keep the legs apart in the Bow Posture. Always start off with the Spinal Rock, which is a warming-up exercise, and conclude by lying a few minutes in the Relaxation Posture, which is described in Chapter 5.

Continue as described in the preceding paragraph for one week, then follow the programme lasting fifteen minutes or that lasting twenty minutes described in Chapter 8. If you are a beginner, you may still need to continue with the simplified variations mentioned above for a few days or weeks. Move to full performance as soon as you are proficient and comfortable in the postures.

After about three months' practice you should start trying out the advanced postures. They may be incorporated into programmes as you become proficient in their practice.

In preparing and practising programmes, please note that any sequence of forward bends should always precede backward bends. The reason for this is that, correctly executed, forward bends straighten the vertebral column and realign it, whereas backward bends tend to exaggerate any distortions in the spine.

Do not exercise within two hours of having a meal.

Your full attention should be given to every moment of each posture – whether going into the posture, staying in it, or coming out of it. In this way practice of the postures becomes an act of meditation or contemplation, calming the mind, in addition to the many psycho-physiological benefits that it produces.

A rug or a folded blanket or something similar should be spread on the floor for comfort. Exercise in a well-ventilated room or outdoors. Remove any belts, ties, or clothing that might constrict or cause discomfort.

# Basic postures

## *Spinal Rock*

This is a warm-up or limber-up exercise. It prepares the body for the stretches of the classic Yoga postures. Students seeking a wider range of limber-up movements may consult *The Complete Yoga Book* (Rider), which describes fifty-five of them.

Lie flat on your back on the floor. Cross your ankles and bring your knees up together on top of your chest. Clasp your arms around your knees. Rounding the back, bring your forehead close to your knees. Rock gently backwards and forwards on the rounded back. Increase the momentum gradually until the soles of the feet are almost touching the floor. Breathe in as you rock forwards and breathe out as you rock backwards.

## Fig. 1   Spinal Rock

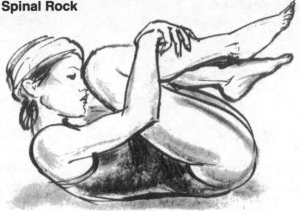

### Benefits

The Spinal Rock massages the spine and the abdomen and removes stiffness in the back. It aids digestion and elimination. It is said to have a beneficial effect on the liver and the spleen.

## *The Tree Posture (Vrksasana)*

Vrksa is a Sanskrit word meaning 'tree'. The traditional Yoga postures or asanas have Sanskrit titles, based on the resemblances of the positions to creatures or objects in nature.

Stand upright. Shift your weight on to the left foot. Fold your right leg and bring your heel up towards the right buttock. Reach back with the right hand and grasp the right foot, pulling it up close to the right buttock. The right and the left thigh should stay in contact. Breathing in, raise your left arm straight up, the upper arm pressing against your left ear. The palm of the left hand faces forward and the fingers point upwards. Balance on the left foot steadily for six seconds at least, then return slowly to the starting position, breathing out. Repeat, balancing on the right leg and raising the right arm. If staying in the pose longer than six seconds start breathing freely.

A more advanced variation is to balance on one leg and place the sole of the foot of the other leg, which is bent, against the inside of the knee of

## Fig 2. Tree Posture

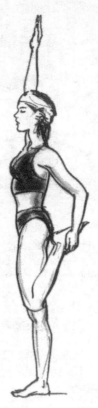

the straight leg. Raise *both* arms and bring the palms of the hands together. Breathe as described above. Repeat, balancing on the other leg.

Balance in both these versions of the Tree Posture is helped by fixing your gaze on the wall in front of you.

### Benefits

The Tree Posture improves balance, posture, poise, and concentration. It deepens the thorax, strengthens the ankles, and firms and tones the muscles of the legs and the trunk. The nervous system benefits from the balancing.

# Triangle Posture (Trikonasana)

Tri means 'three' and kona means 'angle'.

The Tree Posture stretched the body in an upwards direction. The Triangle Posture stretches the body sideways.

Stand upright with your feet widely spaced. Turn out your right foot ninety degrees and your left foot sixty degrees from the midline of the body. Breathing in deeply, extend the arms sideways in line with the shoulders and parallel with the floor, the palms of the hands turned down. Keeping the arms and the legs straight, breathe out and at the same time bend very slowly from the waist sideways to the right, sliding the palm of the right hand as far down the outside of the right leg as it will go. The adept grasps the ankle or the foot, or even places the palm of the hand flat on the floor beside the foot, but the beginner should be satisfied to grasp the calf. As you bend to the right, your straight left arm swings upwards and is held aloft vertically. Twist your head slightly and gaze up at the thumb of your raised left hand. Try to have the two arms in a straight line.

Stay bent over sideways to the right for ten seconds. Breathing in, return very slowly to standing upright in the starting posture in which the arms are extended in line with the shoulders and parallel with the floor. Turn out your left foot ninety degrees and your right foot sixty degrees. Pause five seconds. Exhaling, bend very slowly to the left side, hold the right arm straight up and gaze at the thumb of the right hand, again for ten seconds. Inhaling, return slowly to standing erect. That completes a round. Perform two or three rounds.

## Variations

In a slightly more advanced variation, the head does not move and the arm on the side opposite to that towards which you bend is brought over the head, without bending it, until it presses against the ear and is extended parallel with the floor.

In some variations the legs are spread very far apart and the knee bends on the side to which you are reaching. The other leg stays straight.

The Triangle Posture is a useful posture for beginners in that the degree of stretching can be increased gradually as the body becomes more

**Fig. 3    Triangle Posture**

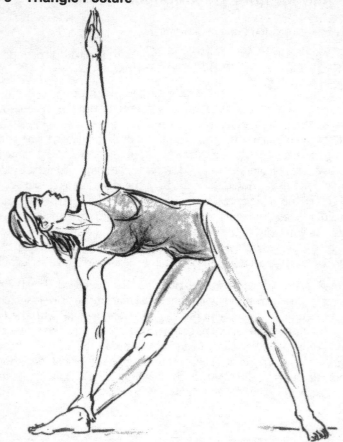

supple. Even if the beginner can only touch the side of the knee, he or she is still benefiting greatly from the posture.

**Benefits**

The Triangle Posture firms and tones the sides and the leg muscles. It is one of the most effective Yoga postures for reducing fat from the waistline. It expands the chest and removes stiffness in the legs and the hips. It stretches and tones the arms, the shoulders, and the back. It massages the abdominal organs. It corrects postural faults.

# The Standing Forward Bend Posture (Padahastasana)

Padahastasana means 'foot-hand posture'. It may be looked upon as the Back-Stretching Posture performed in a standing position. The 'toes touch' exercise we were taught as children has similarities to this Yogic asana. It differs in that you do not perform repetitions of the movement, but hold the pose for at least six seconds. Again the face should be brought as close to the knees as you can comfortably manage, and against the knees in advanced practice.

### Fig. 4   Standing Forward Bend Posture

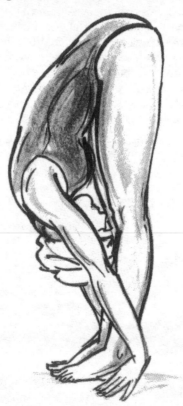

## Benefits

The Standing Forward Bend Posture stretches, strengthens, and limbers the spine. It loosens the 'hamstrings' at the backs of the thighs and firms and tones the legs. It massages the abdominal muscles and viscera. Blood flows to the brain, the scalp, and the facial tissues.

## *The Back-Stretching Posture (Paschimottanasana)*

Paschima means 'back' or 'posterior' and tan means 'stretch'. The back of the body from the heels to the neck is stretched.

This posture has similarities to the well-known 'sit-up' exercise. A number of the exercises popular with physical-culturists in the West have been adapted from Yoga postures. The difference is that in the West the emphasis is on repetition of the movement, whereas in the East the stress is on holding a completed pose without movement. The Back-Stretching Posture differs from a 'sit-up' in another respect; the movement is continued until the face is brought down close to the knees or, in the case of very supple practitioners, actually rests on them.

Lie flat on your back, your legs extended together. Without moving the legs, sit up slowly and smoothly, breathing in. Breathing out, continue

**Fig. 5   Back-Stretching Posture**

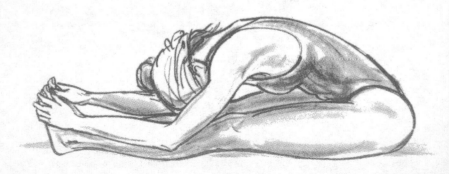

the movement so that your face drops towards your knees. At the same time stretch your arms forward and catch your toes, or your ankles if you cannot reach your feet. Hold the final position for at least six seconds, then slowly bring up your head and upper back, breathing in. If staying bent forward longer than six seconds, breathe freely, taking short breaths.

In all such stretches in Yoga, you should stretch to your limit of comfort, then pause a second or two before easing forward a little further, which you will find you can then do without strain.

### Benefits

The Back-Stretching Posture works the spine in an opposite direction to that of the Cobra Posture and has similar results in promoting its health, strength, and suppleness. It stretches the muscles of the back, the abdomen, the arms and the legs. It aids digestion. It removes surplus fatty tissue from the waistline. It massages the abdomen and its organs.

## The Yoga Headstand (Sirsasana)

Sirsasana means 'head posture' and this is probably one of the best known Yoga postures in the West. Nevertheless, it is in fact an advanced asana that is too strenuous for a great many Westerners, for whom the milder Shoulderstand provides a suitable alternative. It is not suitable for persons suffering from high blood pressure or from diseases of the eye, ears, and brain. If in doubt about the suitability of this posture, seek medical advice. In a Yoga programme, the Headstand should come before the Shoulderstand and Plough Postures, because the Headstand aligns the neck.

Use a thin cushion on a folded towel to protect the top of the head and make sure there is space to roll over if you should overbalance, and a soft surface (a rug or a folded blanket) on which to land. Before starting to learn the Headstand it is advisable to roll over a few times in a relaxed 'ball' so as to take away fear of a fall. Additional security for beginners is to practise in a corner where two walls will provide support for the feet.

The commonest positioning of the hands and arms in the Yoga Headstand is to cup the back of the head with the fingers interlaced and rest the inner

## Fig. 6   Headstand Posture

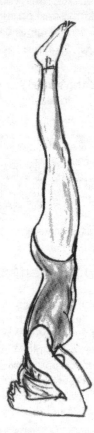

edges of the hands, the forearms and the elbows on the floor. The elbows should not be spread apart more than the width of your shoulders.

The main alternative positioning of the hands is to place the palms on the floor at shoulders' width with the fingers spread apart and pointing forwards, which is the opposite direction to the way you are looking. The weight of the inverted body is then taken on the top of the head and the palms of the hands.

The easiest approach for most students is to bend the knees and bring them in close to the chest. Then take the feet up and over until the soles of the feet face the wall behind the head. The legs are then straightened until the legs, trunk, neck, and head are in a vertical line. Keep the legs and feet relaxed.

Our illustration shows the commonest version in which the hands cup the back of the head and the bodyweight is supported by the inner edges of the hands, the forearms, and the elbows.

More variations of the Headstand and other poses in which the body is inverted may be found in *The Complete Yoga Book* (Rider).

Breathe freely at all stages. Thirty seconds is long enough to hold the inverted position at first, but each week you should be able to add a few seconds until you are comfortable in the topsy-turvy position for several minutes. Progress gradually, ending the posture if you begin to feel any strain. You will probably feel a slight giddiness on returning to standing upright, but this quickly passes.

A simple and non-strenuous way of receiving some of the benefits of Sirsasana is to relax for a few minutes on a board or chair slanted so that the feet are higher than the head.

### Benefits

The customary pull of gravity on the body is reversed in direction. Congestion in the feet, legs, pelvis, and abdomen is eased. Arterial blood flows to the neck, the face, and the brain – hence the posture's reputation for increasing both beauty and intellect. The facial tissues and the roots of the hair are nourished with blood. It refreshes body and mind.

## The Half-Headstand Posture (Ardha-Sirsasana)

Just as there is a Half-Shoulderstand Posture, so too there is a Half-Headstand Posture, practice of which will lead to performance of the full posture.

Kneel with the top of the head on the cushion on the floor and the hands cupping the back of the head with head, hands, forearms, and elbows placed on the floor as described above. It is a fault for the elbows to be placed wider than in line with the shoulders.

## Fig. 7 Half-Headstand Posture

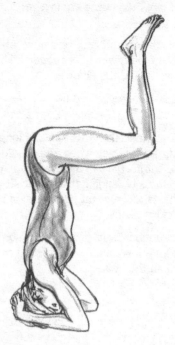

Bend the legs and bring the knees in close to the body by walking forward on the toes from the all-fours position; the knees come inside the elbows and as close to the chest as possible. When the trunk becomes perpendicular and the head, the neck, and the back are in line, support the body firmly on the head, the hands, the forearms, and the elbows and slowly raise the feet together from the floor until the soles of the feet are pointing towards the ceiling with the legs half bent. The lower legs from the knees to the ankles will then be in a vertical position.

Breathe freely throughout all stages. At first stay in the inverted position for only a few seconds, but add seconds as you become accustomed to the pose.

Experience of the Half-Headstand leads in a few weeks to performance of the full Headstand Posture.

## The Shoulderstand Posture (Sarvangasana)

This is sometimes called the All-Body Posture – sarva means 'all' or 'complete' and anga means 'body'. Some writers called it the Candle Posture, because in correct performance the trunk and the legs are perpendicular. There are a variety of shoulderstand postures. It is not suitable for persons with stiff or arthritic necks. Raise the shoulders on something slightly higher than the neck, such as a couple of folded blankets.

Most readers will be familiar with the 'bicycle' exercise, a favourite of athletes and sportsmen, in which you lie on your back and, supporting your hips with your hands, perform a pedalling action with the feet. The Shoulderstand Posture is somewhat similar, but the legs are straightened and the pose is held motionless.

## The Supported Shoulderstand Posture (Salamba Sarvangasana)

Lie flat on your back with your legs stretched out together. Keep the arms close to the sides of the body with the palms of the hands flat on the floor. Bend the legs and bring the knees over the stomach. Lift the hips off the floor and support the right hip with the right hand and the left hip with the left hand. The knees will now be above the chest. Now straighten the trunk and the legs into a vertical position. The hands slide from the hips as the hips are raised and the palms of the hands support the lower back. The thumbs are spread apart from the fingers to give broad support. The chest and the chin press together firmly. The candle-straight trunk and legs are supported by the back of the head and the neck, the shoulders, the backs of the upper arms, and the elbows. The elbows should not be placed wider than the shoulders. Make the necessary adjustment if they are wider than shoulder's width. Do not use the hands any more than is necessary to raise the hips and then maintain balance. The leg muscles and feet should be relaxed. The pose, once you become used to it, should be comfortable.

Breathe freely, into the abdomen, at every stage of the Shoulderstand Posture. This instruction applies to the variations that follow.

— 45 —

## Fig. 8 Supported Shoulderstand Posture

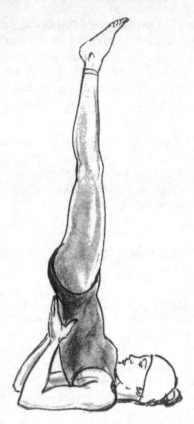

Hold the posture steadily for at least thirty seconds. After a few weeks' practice you should be able to maintain the pose comfortably for from one to five minutes.

Come out of the Shoulderstand slowly by reversing the procedure, returning to lying flat on the back with the legs extended.

### Variations on standard posture

The standard posture described above can be the starting position for several variations. Variations should be looked upon as additions to the standard pose rather than substitutes for it. For example, after staying in the Shoulderstand Posture for about a minute, the legs may be spread apart as far as possible without discomfort, forming a V position which should be maintained for up to thirty seconds. Form the V with the legs three times.

Next spread the legs fore and aft in a slow movement that resembles opening scissors. Again hold the final spread for up to thirty seconds. Then bring the legs together again, pause for about thirty seconds. Then bring the legs together again, pause for about ten seconds, and then repeat the fore and aft 'split', this time reversing the roles of the legs.

## Half-Shoulderstand Posture (Ardha-Sarvangasana)

If you cannot immediately go into the perpendicular posture, then you should begin with the Half-Shoulderstand Posture, in which the legs are straightened above the face at an angle to the floor of about forty-five degrees.

**Fig. 9   Half-Shoulderstand Posture**

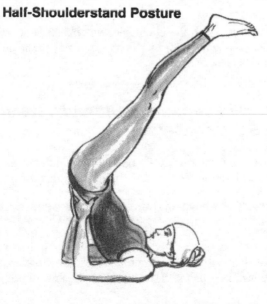

The trunk will slant away at about the same angle, making a right angle approximately between the abdomen and the legs. Support the hips with the hands – the *hips*, not the lower back as in the full Shoulderstand, because the trunk is closer to the floor. Breathe freely into the abdomen. Hold the final position steadily for one to three minutes. Regular practice of the Half-Shoulderstand Posture usually soon leads to the capacity to practise the full Shoulderstand.

## Advanced Supported Shoulderstand Posture (Salamba Sarvangasana)

This advanced posture should not be practised until you are adept in the Shoulderstand Posture in which the hands act as a prop against the lower back, as described above. Go into the propped Shoulderstand, then take the hands from the back and lower them until the palms are flat on the floor and the arms are fully extended along the floor on the opposite side of the body to the head, parallel, shoulders' width apart. The position and direction of the arms is similar to that in the illustration for the Plough Posture. Hold the final position, with the arms straightened, for up to one minute.

In another version, in which the chest receives maximum opening, the arms are extended along the floor on the opposite side of the body to the head and the hands are joined.

## Balancing or Unsupported Shoulderstand (Nirlamba Sarvangasana)

In the most advanced variations of the Shoulderstand Posture, the body balances on the back of the head and the neck, and the shoulders.

In one variation, the hands are taken from the back and the arms are stretched along the floor beyond the head, shoulders' width apart, the palms of the hands turned up. Do not expect the legs to stay vertical; they will tilt slightly over the head. Maintain steadily for up to one minute, breathing freely into the abdomen. In another variation, the body is first supported with the palms of the hands on the lower back, then the

## Fig. 10   Balancing Shoulderstand Posture

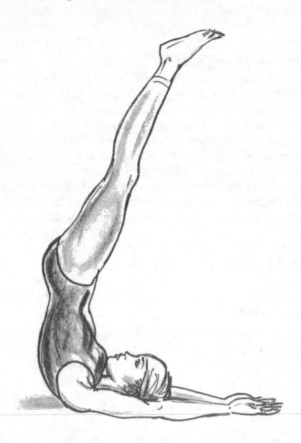

arms are straightened beyond the head and along the floor, the palms of
the hands turned up, as described above. Then raise the arms slowly and
hold the arms upright, so that the palms of the hands are either placed on
the thighs, right palm on the right thigh and left palm on the left thigh, or
alongside the thighs, in which case the thumbs are brought forward so
that the index finger of the right hand is against the side of the right thigh
and the index finger of the left hand is against the side of the left thigh.
Here again, it should be understood that the legs will tilt at a slight angle
above the head. Hold the final position for up to one minute, breathing

freely into the abdomen, as was the instruction for all versions of the Shoulderhand Posture.

**Benefits**

The Shoulderstand Posture benefits every part of the body in some way, so that it is well-named the All-body Posture. It is a milder version of the Yoga Headstand and shares most of its physiological benefits. Blood flows to the brain, the scalp, and the facial tissues. It has a beneficial effect on the endocrine glands, in particular the thyroid and parathyroid glands. It stretches and strengthens the spine. The muscles of the legs, back, abdomen, and neck are also stretched. It soothes and tones the nervous system. It releases congestion in the legs, pelvis, and abdomen. It relieves and prevents varicose veins in the legs. It reduces excess fat. It improves the health of the organs of the pelvis and the abdomen, and it is said to increase sexual fitness in both men and women.

## *Plough Posture (Halasana)*

Hala is the Sanskrit word for 'plough'. Traditionally, the Yoga postures (asanas) have Sanskrit names.

The Plough Posture follows naturally out of the preceding Shoulderstand Posture and may be made a continuation of it. If in the Shoulderstand Posture you swing over your feet and legs until the toes touch the floor

**Fig. 11   Plough Posture**

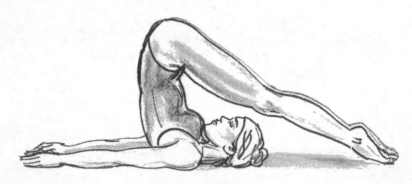

behind the head you will be in the Plough Posture. The hands are taken from the lower back and the palms are pressed down flat on the floor with the arms extended, at shoulders' width apart, on the opposite side of the body to the head. Your legs should be together and straightened out. When the toes touch the ground, attempt to push them as far as possible towards the wall behind the head.

The resemblance of the final position to the shape of an Indian plough gave this asana its name.

Beginners find that the feet at first do not reach the floor, but usually they do so with a little practice. Be patient and avoid straining. Forcing the feet to touch the floor behind the head may strain the neck muscles: the feet should drop effortlessly to the floor. Stay steadily in the final position for at least six seconds, increasing the number of seconds gradually as the posture becomes more comfortable.

Breathe as freely as the pose allows, taking short rapid breaths through the nostrils.

Beginners may wish to support the back with the hands in the first few weeks before going on to the unsupported posture.

**Note:** This pose is not suitable for persons with weak vertebrae.

### Benefits

The Plough Posture keeps the spine supple and youthful and helps maintain its natural curve. It tones the nervous system and stretches and makes more supple almost all the body muscles. It stimulates the endocrine glands, the liver and the spleen. It corrects menstrual disorders and is said to enhance sexual fitness. It massages the abdomen and prevents disorders of the stomach, and is also one of the best postures for normalising the obese figure.

## The Cobra Posture (Bhujangasana)

Bhujanga means 'cobra'. The posture resembles a cobra about to strike.

Lie flat on the abdomen with your chest on the floor. The arms are bent and the palms of the hands rest on the floor close in to the shoulders. The

## Fig. 12  Cobra Posture

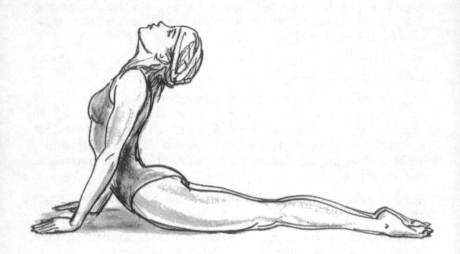

fingers point forwards. Keep the elbows in against the sides of the body. Your forehead should also be touching the floor and your legs are fully extended and kept together throughout the pose.

Slowly raise your head upwards and backwards. The face, the neck, and the trunk will follow gradually. The spine bends vertebra by vertebra. In the final position, which should be held motionless, the arms are straight or almost so and the head is thrown back so that the eyes look at an angle towards the ceiling.

The important thing in performing this exercise is to put as much work as possible on to the spine. You will probably find that you have to use your arms to help you – indeed at first they will be doing most of the work. With practice, however, it is possible for some people to dispense altogether with the aid of the arms.

Remember that the movement should be slow and smooth, with no jerking or straining. The spine must be treated with great care. Inhale as you slowly raise the head, neck, and upper back successively. The legs and the pelvis remain in contact with the floor. On reaching the Cobra-about-to-strike position, stay motionless for six seconds. Breathe out as you return slowly to the starting position lying face down on the floor. If holding the pose for longer than six seconds, start breathing freely after six seconds.

## Variations

Some instructors favour keeping as much of the abdomen as possible in contact with the floor, ideally up to the navel. Only adepts can do this and straighten the arms. Hence some teachers instruct their pupils to straighten their arms only so far as raising the trunk allows without the abdomen lifting off the floor.

There is a simplified beginner's variation in which the palms of the hands are placed on the floor, the fingers pointing forwards, some five to six inches in front of the shoulders, the width of the shoulders apart – not close in to the shoulders, as taught above. This permits easier back-bending, the arms are easier to straighten, and more of the abdomen stays in contact with the floor. As proficiency increases in this exercise, the hands may be gradually brought closer to the shoulders, until finally they are close in to them.

## Benefits

The Cobra Posture curves the spine inwards, vertebra by vertebra, from the lumbar region to the neck. The front of the body is stretched. The throat and jawline are firmed. It reduces abdominal fat. It strengthens the spine and increases its suppleness. It improves the efficiency of the nervous system. It improves body metabolism. It corrects faulty posture.

## *The Bow Posture (Dhanurasana)*

Dhanu means 'bow'. The pose resembles a drawn bow.

Lie flat on your stomach. Stretch your arms back and, raising the heels, grasp both ankles. Pulling with your arms, lift the legs as high as possible, at the same time arching the front part of the body. It is as if you were trying to touch the back of your head with the soles of your feet.

Breathe freely. Hold the drawn-bow position for at least six seconds.

This pose is not easy at first and beginners usually have to keep their legs a little apart. As the muscles strengthen, the legs should be brought closer together until finally they can be kept in contact throughout performance.

### Benefits

The Bow Posture stretches and strengthens the spine and makes it more supple. It stretches the muscles of the abdomen, the back, the legs, the arms and the neck. It tones the nervous system. It improves the efficiency of the liver, the kidneys and the glands. It improves digestion. It is one of the finest correctives for faulty posture.

**Fig. 13    Bow Posture**

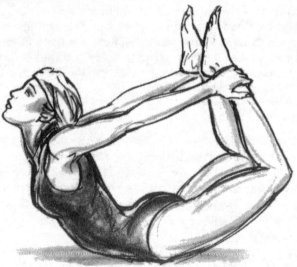

## *The Thunderbolt Posture (Vajrasana)*

Vajra means 'thunderbolt'. This pose is sometimes called the Adamantor Adamantine Posture. A number of important Yogic postures use the Thunderbolt Posture as their starting position.

Kneel with the legs together and the buttocks resting on the feet, the soles of which are upturned. Rest the palm of the right hand on the right knee and the palm of the left hand on the left knee. The head is held erect and the back straight.

Pain in the knee-joints should go away with regular practice. Breathe freely and deeply into the abdomen. Sit motionless for at least thirty seconds.

**Fig. 14   Thunderbolt Posture**

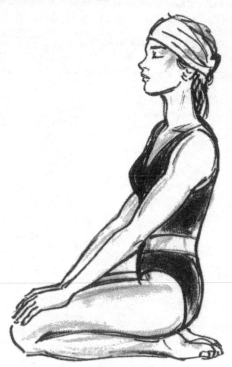

## Benefits

Sitting in the Thunderbolt Posture calms the nervous system and quietens the mind. It improves posture. It firms and tones the legs and limbers the knee-joints. It stimulates digestion. It encourages healthful deep abdominal breathing. It makes a suitable posture for breathing exercises for the person who cannot sit correctly in one of the cross-legged positions.

## The Lion Posture (Simhasana)

Simha means 'lion'. This posture is one of many which is based on the Thunderbolt position. Sit on your heels with the back straight and the head and the back in a vertical line. The arms are extended so that the left palm rests on the left knee and the right palm is placed on the right knee.

Exhaling, straighten the arms and tense the whole body. Open the eyes and the mouth widely and protrude the tongue out and down as far as possible. Sustain the contraction for six seconds. Let go and breathe in.

**Fig. 15　Lion Posture**

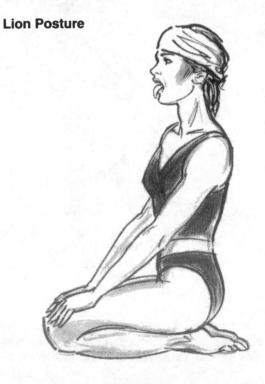

**Benefits**

The Lion Posture brings blood to the throat and the larynx and to the facial muscles. The face – the most important and expressive set of muscles we possess – tends to be neglected in exercise programmes. Yoga, in its wisdom, takes the facial muscles into account. For a full programme of exercises to improve the contours and health of the face and the neck, see *New Faces* (Thorsons).

## The Cowface Posture (Gomukhasana)

Go means 'cow' and mukha means 'face'.

This is usually performed in the Thunderbolt position, though it may also be performed in any sitting or standing posture in which the back is kept straight and upright.

**Fig. 16   Cowface Posture**

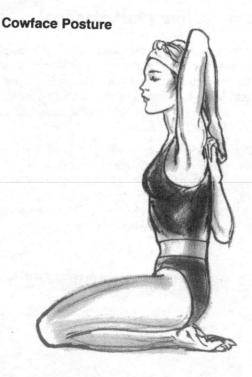

Bend the right arm, raise the elbow high and stretch the hand over the right shoulder and down the centre of the back as far as you can reach without disturbing the straight line of the spine. At the same time bend the left arm and bring the left hand up the back until the fingers of the two hands meet and lock together at the fingertips. The palm of the right hand is facing the back and the palm of the left hand is facing outwards. Breathing freely, stay in the pose at least six seconds. Repeat, reversing the arm positions.

### Benefits

The Cowface Posture improves posture, limbers the shoulder joints, strengthens and tones the muscles of the upper back and those of the upper arms. This is an excellent corrective exercise for people with sedentary occupations.

## The Mountain Posture (Parbatasana)

Sit in one of the postures for meditation (see p. 67). In the simplest of the cross-legged postures, the Easy Posture, you sit on the floor, keeping the head and the back in a straight vertical line, and cross the legs in what is sometimes called tailor's sitting. Persons who find even the Easy Posture uncomfortable may sit on a straight-backed chair or a stool, keeping the soles of the feet flat on the floor.

Now stretch both arms towards the ceiling and bring the palms of the hands and the fingers together directly above your head as in the attitude of prayer. Then stretch your fingertips straight upwards as far as they will go comfortably. Sit without moving for at least twenty seconds, breathing slowly and deeply into the abdomen. The pose should have the solid immovability of a mountain (parbat).

### Benefits

The stretching action benefits the muscles of the trunk and the abdomen, strengthens the spine, tones the nervous system, improves digestion and corrects constipation. The abdominal breathing purifies the bloodstream and calms the mind.

**Fig. 17   Mountain Posture**

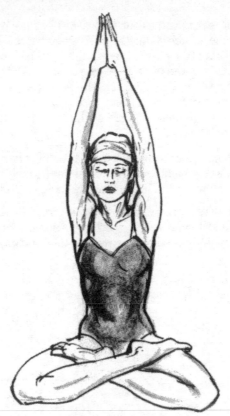

## ———— Advanced postures ————

I now give some of the best known of the postures requiring either considerable suppleness or strength. For most students they will be targets to aim for – though the student should not be greatly disappointed if most or even all of them are unattainable, for the preceding postures provide an ample basis for highly beneficial programmes. Once any of the advanced postures allow comfortable performance they can be fitted into a daily programme.

## *The Twist Posture (Ardha-Matsyendrasana)*

Sit on the floor with your legs outstretched. Bend the right leg and place its heel into the crotch as in the first stage of the Perfect Posture (Chapter 6). Bring the left foot across the right leg and place it on the floor outside it. With the right hand, grasp the toes of the left foot from outside the left knee. The trunk and the head are twisted round to do this, and the free left arm is bent across the lower back with the palm of the left hand facing outwards. This works the spine from a new angle, since it is twisted laterally.

Hold the pose for a few seconds at first, breathing freely, adding to the time gradually as the body becomes accustomed to the position. Perform the twist to the opposite side to complete the exercise.

Patience and perseverance may bring success in this posture, but persons who find it impossible can achieve a somewhat similar effect by sitting on a straight-backed chair, twisting round and grasping the ends of

**Fig. 18　Twist Posture**

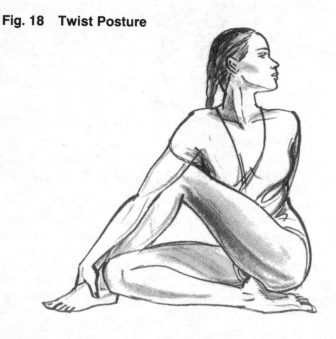

the chair back with both hands. Keep the legs and the hips steady. Twist the head and the trunk right round as far as they will go without strain.

### Benefits

The Twist Posture benefits the nervous system, the stomach, the kidneys and the liver.

## The Knee and Head Posture (Janusirasana)

This may be viewed as a one-legged Back-Stretching Posture.

Sit on the floor with your legs together and outstretched. Bending the left leg at the knee, grasp the left ankle and pull the heel in against the crotch, as for the Perfect Posture (see p. 79). The right leg is kept fully stretched. Exhaling, lean forward slowly and grasp your right foot with both hands. Still breathing out, lower your head between your arms and attempt to touch your right knee with your head. Very supple people will be able to to so.

Sustain the bent forward position for six seconds at least, then sit up slowly; breathing in. If staying down longer than six seconds, breathe freely after six seconds.

Repeat, bending the right leg and leaning forward to grasp the left foot.

### Fig. 19   Knee and Head Posture

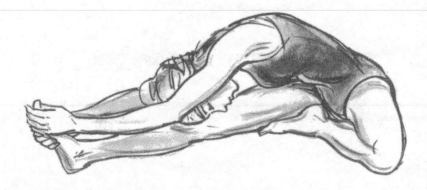

**Benefits**

The Knee and Head Posture benefits the whole body, making the spine more supple and strengthening the spinal nerves. The abdomen is squeezed and surplus fat is removed from the waistline.

## The Yoga Posture (Yogasana)

Sit in the Lotus Posture, in which each foot is upturned on the opposite thigh (see p. 80). The arms are placed behind the back with the right hand grasping the left wrist, or the left hand grasping the right wrist. Exhale and lean forward to touch the floor with your forehead, or as near to the floor as you can lower the head.

Stay in the bent forward position for at least twenty seconds, breathing freely. The pose has a compact beauty when successfully performed. It is sometimes called the Symbol of Yoga (Yoga Mudra).

**Benefits**

The Yoga Posture benefits the abdomen in both the external muscles and the internal organs, which are squeezed. The back is stretched along its full length. This posture is said to correct constipation, stomach disorders and obesity.

**Fig. 20  Yoga Posture**

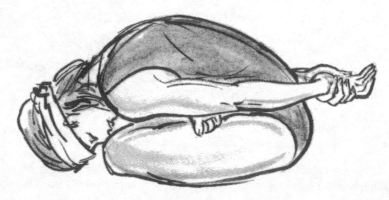

## *The Locust Posture (Salabhasana)*

Lie flat and full length on your abdomen, your chin resting on the floor, and your hands, palms up, resting on the floor beside your hips. The legs are extended and together. Taking a deep breath, raise the legs as high as possible. If you succeed, the action resembles that of a locust. More height can be gained by bringing the hands together, making fists, beneath the groin. Experts raise the legs, pelvis, abdomen, and lower chest clear of the floor. You press down with your arms and the lower back muscles do most of the work. Hold the legs-raised position for several seconds, then, exhaling, lower the legs slowly to the floor.

### Benefits

This is a vigorous exercise, benefiting the abdomen and the lower back. Most beginners will need to perform the Half-Locust Posture for a time before tackling the full Locust Posture.

### Fig. 21   Locust Posture

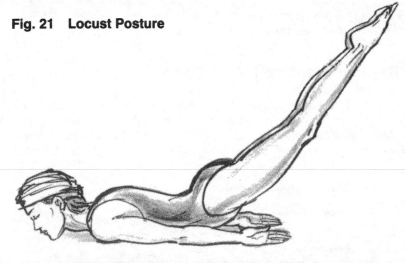

## *The Half-Locust Posture (Ardha-Salabhasana)*

You lie face down as before, with your chin on the floor but instead of raising both legs you raise the left and right legs separately. Take a deep

## Fig. 22   Half-Locust Posture

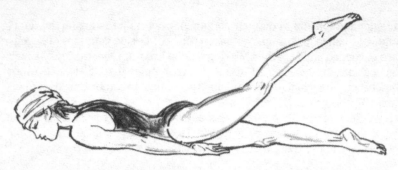

breath as you raise a leg and exhale as you lower it slowly. Keep the leg raised as high as possible for several seconds.

### Benefits

The benefits are similar in nature to those for full performance, but the effects are much milder.

## *The Fish Posture (Matsyasana)*

First sit cross-legged in the Lotus Posture (see p. 80), then lean back until the body is supported by the top of the head. Hold your right foot, which is upturned on the left thigh, with the right hand, and hold the left foot, which is upturned on the right thigh, with the right hand. Inhale

### Fig. 23   Fish Posture

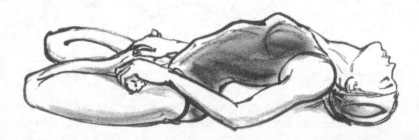

deeply, expanding the chest. The back should be fully arched and the chest spread out.

In this posture you can float easily on the sea, hence its name The Fish Posture. There is some similarity to the 'Wrestler's Bridge' of Western physical-culture.

**Benefits**

The neck, the brain, the chest, the spine and the stomach all benefit.

## The Supine Thunderbolt Posture (Supta-Vajrasana)

Sit on your heels with your knees together in the Thunderbolt Posture. Keeping the legs still, slowly bend backwards. Most people will at first need to employ the arms and the elbows as an aid to lowering the trunk. Lower the shoulders until they rest firmly on the floor. Then stretch your arms full length beyond your head, with the palms of your hands turned upwards.

Hold the supine posture for at least twenty seconds, increasing the time gradually as the body becomes accustomed to the stretch.

**Benefits**

The supine Thunderbolt Posture has a health-giving stretching action on the thighs and the stomach. It prevents constipation and aids digestion. It enlarges the rib-cage and removes excess flab.

**Fig. 24   Supine Thunderbolt Posture**

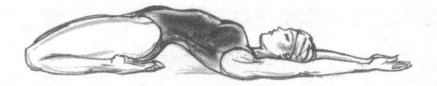

## *The Wheel Posture (Chakrasana)*

Lie flat on your back on the floor. Bending your knees, draw your heels in against your buttocks. At the same time bend your arms and place the palms of your hands on the floor on either side of your head, with your fingers pointing back towards your heels. To do this you will probably have to raise your buttocks a little. Distribute your bodyweight on the soles of your feet and the palms of your hands. Now raise your trunk upwards until the feet and the hands take the full strain and the back is fully arched.

'The Wheel' will be familiar to keen gymnasts. It is a strenuous exercise and should only be attempted by advanced practitioners.

### Benefits

The Wheel Posture strengthens the spine and the nervous system, prevents and cures abdominal disorders, and reduces surplus fat. The whole front of the body is powerfully stretched.

**Fig. 25   The Wheel**

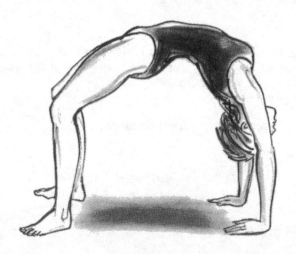

## *The Peacock Posture (Mayurasana)*

This is a vigorous exercise that will appeal to gymnasts.

Commence from a kneeling position with the knees spread apart. Place the palms of the hands together on the floor with the fingers pointing towards your feet. The wrists should be touching. Lean forward on the hands with the elbows resting against the stomach. Now bring the bodyweight forward and straighten the legs until the body balances on the hands and the elbows in a straight line parallel to the floor. Exhale as you lean forward to start balancing, but make short rapid breaths as you balance for as many seconds as you find comfortable.

### Benefits

The Peacock Posture massages and strengthens the abdominal area.

### Fig. 26   Peacock Posture

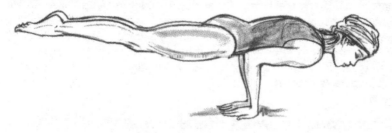

## —— The postures of meditation ——

The best-known standard asanas have been described in this chapter. However, there are four more asanas which cannot be omitted from any work on Hatha Yoga. The first three are the sitting positions for meditation, for breathing exercises, and for performance of many asanas. They are Easy Posture (Sukhasana), Perfect Posture (Siddhasana) and Lotus Posture (Padmasana). They will be described in Chapter 6 on Yoga breathing.

The fourth asana is the Relaxation or Corpse Posture (Savasana). The need for relaxation being so great in the West, a separate chapter (5) will be given to this subject.

Also, Chapter 8 describes the Yoga Cat Stretch which is a combination of several postures and is useful when time is strictly limited.

## 8,400,000 Asanas

In the *Gheranda Samhita*, a key Sanskrit text on Hatha Yoga, we read that 'there are eighty-four hundreds of thousands of asanas described by Siva. The postures are as many in number as there are living creatures in this universe.' This is, of course, an exaggeration to which such classic texts are prone. The *Gheranda Samhita* goes on to say that 'eighty-four are the best' and among these 'thirty-two have been found useful for mankind in this world'. The best-known standard asanas have been described in this chapter. There are, however, other Indian postures and a wealth of variations and adaptations of classic Indian postures that are now practised in the West. All of these, together with warm-up and limber-up exercises essential for most Westerners starting Yoga, are described and illustrated in *The Complete Yoga Book* (Rider). The total number of postures described is four hundred and eighteen. Guidance is also given for compiling programmes for beginners, intermediate and advanced students.

## Therapeutic powers of the asanas

Therapeutic powers are claimed for the asanas. The work of such institutions as the Yoga Research Laboratory at Lonavla has done much to give these claims a scientific basis. Below I list some common disorders and the postures and muscle controls given in this book which are said by Yoga experts to provide a relief or cure. However, the postures are not suggested as a substitute for medical care.

Most of the postures listed are described in this chapter but the Easy, Perfect and Lotus Postures are found in Chapter 6 on Yoga breathing, the two cleansing exercises (Abdominal Retraction and Isolation of the Recti Muscles) in Chapter 7, and the Yoga Cat Stretch in Chapter 8.

## Asthma

Fish, Locust, Mountain, Relaxation, Shoulderstand.

## Backache

Back-stretching, Cat, Cowface, Fish, Headstand, Plough, Relaxation, Shoulderstand, Supine Thunderbolt, Tree.

## Bronchitis

Cobra, Fish, Locust, Lotus, Mountain, Shoulderstand.

## Constipation

Abdominal Retraction, Back-stretching, Fish, Forward Bend, Headstand, Head-Knee, Plough, Bow, Recti Isolation, Shoulderstand, Twist, Yoga.

## Diabetes

Back-stretching, Cobra, Peacock, Plough, Relaxation, Shoulderstand, Twist, Yoga.

## Indigestion

Abdominal Retraction, Cobra, Mountain, Peacock, Plough, Recti Isolation, Relaxation, Shoulderstand, Supine Thunderbolt, Yoga.

## Insomnia

Back-stretching, Cobra, Locust, Mountain, Plough, Relaxation, Shoulderstand.

## Lumbago

Locust, Plough, Relaxation, Tree, Twist.

## Menopause Disorders

Abdominal Retraction, Cat, Cobra, Fish, Plough, Relaxation, Shoulderstand, sitting postures.

## Menstrual Disorders

Abdominal Retraction, Back-stretching, Cat, Cobra, Fish, Forward Bend, Headstand, Head-Knee, Plough, Recti Isolation, Relaxation, Shoulderstand, sitting postures.

## Neurasthenia

Back-stretching, Headstand, Mountain, Relaxation, Shoulderstand, Tree, Yoga.

## Obesity

Abdominal Retraction, Back-stretching, Bow, Cobra, Forward Bend, Head-Knee, Plough, Triangle, Twist.

## Piles

Fish, Headstand, Plough, Shoulderstand.

## Rheumatism

Back-stretching, Bow, Cowface, Knee and Head, Twist, Triangle.

## Sexual Debility

Abdominal Retraction, Bow, Cat, Cobra, Headstand, Plough, Recti Isolation, Shoulderstand, all the sitting and kneeling postures, Twist, Yoga.

## Tension

Abdominal Retraction, Back-stretching, Forward Bend, Mountain, Relaxation, Shoulderstand, Tree, Triangle.

## Varicose Veins

Headstand, Shoulderstand.

Yoga breathing also has therapeutic powers and has particular relevance in the following disorders: Asthma, backache, bronchitis, constipation, insomnia, menopause and menstrual disorders, neurasthenia, obesity, sexual debility, tension.

# 5

# — YOGA RELAXATION —

Western civilised man lives at a pace that would have left his forefathers breathless and bewildered. His nervous system is subject to almost constant strain. Under the stress of such a way of life it is not surprising that his health is usually below par and that diseases and complaints resulting from tension have become so prevalent. It has been estimated that at least fifty per cent of the people who visit doctors' consulting rooms suffer from neurasthenia rather than from any organic disorder.

One of the immediate benefits reported by people taking up Yoga is that they feel more relaxed. This is a natural result of sitting still in the asanas, of breath control, thought control and meditation. Yoga quickly calms the mind, relaxes the body.

## The relaxation posture

While all the eight limbs of Yoga have a relaxing influence, the Yogi usually finishes his programme of asanas with one especially designed to rest the body and re-charge it with energy.

This is Savasana, the Relaxation or Corpse Posture. It is of such value in

## Fig. 27  Relaxation or 'Corpse' Posture

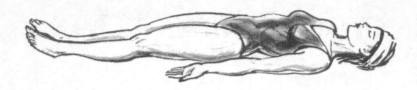

combating present-day stress and strain that you should perform it at any time you can during the day.

Lie flat on your back with your legs outstretched. Close your eyes and remain completely still, as if dead. This means lying with your full weight. You must really 'let go'.

You cannot expect to attain complete relaxation at the first attempt. It is an art which has to be mastered and this may take weeks, even months. But all the time you will be benefiting.

At first you will find that an obstinate tension remains and the body muscles refuse to relax. You must mentally go over them from head to toe seeking tension and removing it wherever it is found. Follow a definite order in relaxing the various muscles and muscle groups. This order is given below.

**The scalp and the forehead**
**The eyes and the eyeballs**
**The jaw and the mouth**
**The throat**
**The neck**
**The trapezius** (across the top of the back, below the neck)
**The deltoids** (shoulders)
**The latissimus dorsi** (the two large wedge-shaped muscles covering the shoulder-blades)
**The abdomen**
**The pectorals** (the breasts)
**The triceps** (the rear parts of the upper arms)

**The biceps** (the front parts of the upper arms)
**The forearms**
**The hands and the fingers**
**The buttocks**
**The biceps of the thighs** (the rear parts of the thighs)
**The extensors of the thighs** (the front parts of the thighs)
**The calves**
**The feet and the toes**

Having taken your awareness on a journey over the whole body from the scalp to the toes, do so again in reverse order. Seek out tension and release it in each of the nineteen muscle groups, starting with the feet and moving up the body until reaching the forehead and the scalp.

The ability to relax comes more quickly if you can 'get the feel' of all nineteen muscles or muscle groups by alternately tensing and relaxing them. In this way you learn to 'talk' to your muscles. Special muscle control exercises for achieving this are given in my book *Relaxation* in the Teach Yourself series.

For the Relaxation Posture it is best to lie on the floor on a folded blanket. Collars, ties and other constricting clothing should be removed. You cannot relax if you feel uncomfortable in any way.

As you become more adept you will find that you will be able to relax with a fair degree of success even in a sitting position, a neuro-muscular skill which you can utilise in travelling by bus or train to and from your place of employment.

There is no more efficacious way of combating tension than to have a daily relaxation period or periods. So from now on make it a rule to perform the Relaxation Posture (Savasana) at least once every day.

# 6

## YOGA BREATHING (PRANAYAMA)

Pranayama – from prana (the life breath) and ayama (pause) – is the Yoga science of breath control.

The ancient Yogis studied anatomy and explored body and consciousness to learn their secrets. One of the important things they discovered was the reciprocal relationship between the emotions and breathing. When we are excited our rate of respiration becomes faster. When we are composed, our breathing is slow, calm and rhythmical. The Yogi seeks, by controlled and measured breathing, to influence consciousness itself. By control of the breath the mind can be stilled and made one-pointed. Pranayama is a means to self-mastery and psychic powers.

## Prana

It is necessary to point out that Prana, to the Yogi, means much more than mere breath. Prana is actually the power both behind and within breath. The power of the atom is Prana. Thought is Prana. It is 'the vital force in every being'. It is cosmetic energy. It pervades the whole universe. It is everywhere and through Pranayama we can tap this illimitable well of universal energy.

Vivekananda, in his *Raja Yoga*, says:

> In this body of ours the breath motion is the 'silken thread'; by laying hold of and learning to control it we grasp the pack thread of the nerve currents, and from these the stout twine of our thoughts, and lastly the rope of Prana, controlling which we reach freedom.

We do not know anything about our own bodies; we cannot know. At best we can take a dead body, and cut it in pieces, and there are some who can take a live animal and cut it in pieces in order to see what is inside the body. Still, that has nothing to do with our own bodies. We know very little about them. Why do we not? Because our attention is not discriminating enough to catch the very fine movements that are going on within. We can know of them only when the mind becomes more subtle and enters, as it were, deeper into the body. To get that subtle perception we have to begin with the grosser perceptions. We have to get hold of that which is setting the whole engine in motion; that is the Prana, the most obvious manifestation of which is the breath. Then along with the breath, we shall slowly enter the body, which will enable us to find out about the subtle forces, the nerve currents that are moving all over the body. As soon as we perceive and learn to feel them, we shall begin to get control over them, and over the body. The mind is also set in motion by these different nerve currents, so at last we shall reach the state of perfect control over the body and the mind, making both our servants. Knowledge is power; we have to get this power, so we must begin at the beginning, the Pranayama, restraining the Prana.

## *Breath is life*

To prepare the mind for the meditative exercises and disciplines, the Yogi seeks to control respiration, the body's key function and 'the most obvious manifestation of Prana'. Life is impossible without air. We can do without food and water for several days, but totally check our air supply and we are dead in a few minutes.

Our bodies need oxygen to burn up waste matter and to purify the bloodstream. Civilised man has lost the art of breathing properly. His shallow breathing utilises only about one-tenth of his lung capacity. The lack of oxygen from which he inevitably suffers is responsible for headaches, fatigue, lack of mental alertness. It is a contributory cause of that 'tired feeling' so many people complain of today. (A yawn is Nature's way of enabling us to get more oxygen when there is a lack of it.)

The Yoga breathing exercises, if performed sensibly and without strain, can be a means to greater bodily vitality, and can exert a beneficial influence over the emotions and the mind.

# The meditative postures

For Pranayama and meditation the Yogis use certain seated postures which keep the body compact and perfectly steady. The three best known of these are the Easy Posture (Sukhasana), the Perfect Posture (Siddhasana) and the Lotus Posture (Padmasana). They provide rock-like and symmetrical stability, combined with alert poise.

These seated postures are familiar to the Oriental from childhood, but the Occidental, more accustomed to sitting on chairs, may find that his joints are too stiff to perform them at first or he may find them uncomfortable and painful. Do not use force: some Westerners, impatient for progress, have damaged their knees. Sitting on a cushion enables the position to be adopted more easily. One method of preparatory training is to sit on the floor and bend one leg only. Grasp the ankle and pull the foot in against the perineum, the soft flesh between the anus and the scrotum or vulva. Keep the other leg extended. Stay in that position for two or three minutes, then repeat with the other leg. Do this a few times. Later you should perform the preparatory training with a view to achieving the Lotus Posture. Instead of taking the foot in against the perineum, upturn it on the opposite thigh high up against the groin. Again each leg should be bent alternately and the other leg kept fully extended. Place the palms of the hands on the floor level with the hips to prevent overbalancing backwards.

## Egyptian Posture

Persons who, for whatever reason, cannot use the cross-legged postures, may perform the breathing exercises or meditate while sitting on a straightbacked chair. The important thing is for the body to be perfectly steady with the head, the neck and the back in a straight line. Rest the palms of the hands flat on the thighs, the left hand on the left thigh and the right hand on the right thigh. The position resembles that seen in some Egyptian statues. It has some of the advantages of the cross-legged postures, but it is worth making the effort to master the latter.

**Fig. 28  Egyptian Posture**

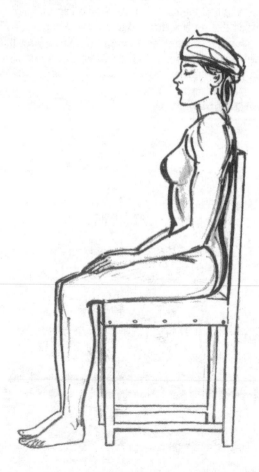

## *Easy Posture (Sukhasana)*

This is within the capacity of most beginners. When you can lower your knees to the floor and stay there for at least ten minutes without discomfort, it will be time to move on to the more advanced Perfect and Lotus postures.

Sit on the floor with both legs extended. Now bend one leg and place the foot under the thigh of the other leg. Then bend that leg and place the foot under the other leg. At first your knees will probably stay up off the floor, but in time you will be able to lower them. You should aim eventually to place your knees flat on the floor. Meanwhile keep your knees widely spaced and as close to the ground as possible. Keep your back erect and straight, though not rigidly so, with the head in line with the back and hold the chin level. The choice of positions for the hands will be described

**Fig. 29   Easy Posture**

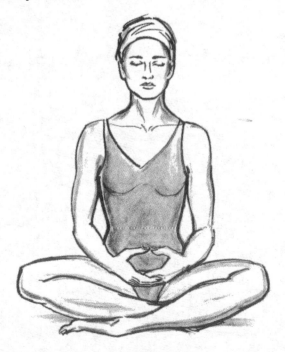

shortly. Though the Easy Posture has not the full stability of the Perfect and Lotus Postures, it is possible nevertheless to experience something of the poise and symmetry that make the cross-legged postures so satisfactory for meditation. Their advantage for breathing exercises is their steadiness and the freedom given to the diaphragm and the other muscles of respiration.

Vary the order in which you cross your legs. Sometimes draw in the right leg before the left and at other times draw in the left leg first.

## *Perfect Posture (Siddhasana)*

The preparatory training for this has already been discussed. Bend the left leg and, grasping the ankle, draw the left foot in against the perineum

**Fig. 30   Perfect Posture**

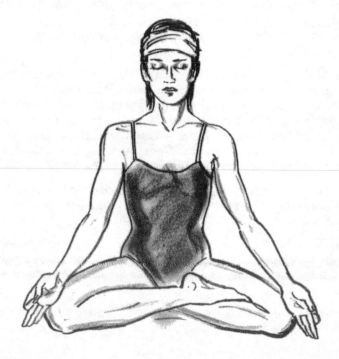

(between the anus and the scrotum or vulva). The right leg is then bent and the foot drawn in towards the body and placed in the crevice between the calf and the thigh of the left leg with the heel against the pubic bone.

Again the head, the neck, and the back should be in a straight vertical line. Both knees are on the ground and, by resting the hands or wrists on the knees or cupping the hands in the lap, perfect stability and symmetry can be attained and experienced.

Vary the order in which you cross your legs so that sometimes the right foot is in against the perineum and sometimes the left foot.

## Lotus Posture (Padmasana)

This is the most famous of the Eastern postures for meditation. It is seen in statues of the serene meditating Buddha. Most Westerners find it difficult and many never manage it. Others manage it after weeks or months of increasing flexibility. Preparatory training has already been described, in which one foot is upturned on the opposite thigh and one leg is kept fully extended. There is, too, a Half-Lotus Posture which may be used prior to use of the full Lotus Posture.

Sit on the floor with both legs extended. Bend one leg, grasp the ankle, and pull the foot in against the perineum, as for the Perfect Posture. The knee is flat on the floor. Now bend the other leg, grasp the ankle, and draw the foot up high on the thigh of the other leg as near as possible to the groin. At first the knee may stay obstinately off the floor, but with practice you will be able to lower it. Once both knees are on the floor and you can sustain the posture easily, move on to the full Lotus Posture.

Alternate the roles of the legs. Keep the left foot on the right thigh for a few minutes and then place the right foot on the left thigh for a few minutes.

In the full Lotus Posture the right foot is on the left thigh and the left foot is on the right thigh. Once you are comfortable in the Lotus Posture it provides maximum poise and stability for breathing exercises or for meditation.

Sometimes cross the left leg over the right and sometimes cross the right leg over the left.

**Fig. 31   Lotus Posture**

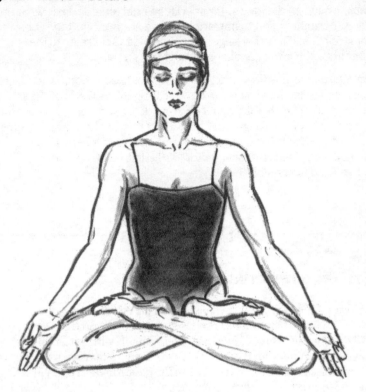

## *Thunderbolt Posture (Vajrasana)*

Some people use the Thunderbolt Posture, in which you sit on your heels the way the Japanese do, for practising Pranayama. It was described in Chapter 4. Here again the back may be kept straight and the respiratory muscles function freely.

## *Hand positions*

The placing of the hands in these sitting postures has not been mentioned. Several positions are possible.

One of the oldest traditional positions is with the wrists, either front or back, placed on the knees, right wrist on right knee and left wrist on left knee. Forefinger and thumb are bent and are brought together to form rough circles. The other fingers are extended. According to the length of your arm, the arms are almost straight or straight.

An alternative position, which is restful for meditation, is to place the back of your left hand on the palm of your right hand and have both hands in your lap. The thumbs either overlap, left over right, or are brought together to form a rough oval. In Perfect Posture or Lotus Posture the back of the right hand may rest on an upturned heel. If you are left-handed, rest the right hand on top of the left hand. The idea is that the active hand is immobilised.

# Pranayama

## Pre-requirements

Before commencing Pranayama it is required that the body should be clean and free of impurities. Have a sponge down and clear your nostrils by blowing each separately. Rinse your mouth with water and rub your tongue and gums with the fingers. Some readers may wish to sniff water through the nostrils and expel it from the mouth in the Yogic cleansing act called Neti (see Chapter 7, page 89).

At least two hours should have elapsed since a meal.

The exercises should be performed in the open, before an open window, or at least in an airy room.

Wear loose fitting clothes, but don't risk catching cold. Remove constricting collars and ties.

## The Cleansing Breath (Kapalabhati)

Kapalabhati is now usually included in Pranayama practice, though it is one of the six purification practices (see Chapter 2). It is designed to clear the sinuses and rid the nerve channels (nadis) of impurities and should precede the other breathing exercises.

As with all the breathing exercises given in this chapter it is best performed in one of the meditative postures.

Inhalation (puraka) and exhalation (rechaka) take place through the nose, the latter being accomplished by means of a quick and vigorous contraction of the abdominal muscles and diaphragm.

Take a deep breath through both nostrils and then retract the abdominal muscles and diaphragm in a sharp instroke that forces the air out of your nose so fast as to be almost a sneeze. Immediately the exhalation is finished, inhale again.

Exhalation should take less time than inhalation. At the start do it ten times at the rate of two exhalations per second. This completes a round. Take a minute's rest, breathing normally, before commencing a further round.

You should be able to add to the size of a round until you are doing twenty or more inhalations and exhalations. Speed too can be increased but this should never be at the expense of efficiency.

There is likely to be a slight soreness of the abdomen at first until the muscles strengthen. Daily practice of Uddiyana as described in Chapter 7 will facilitate the performance of Kapalabhati.

### Benefits

Cleansing Breath clears the nasal passages and cleanses the sinuses. It enriches the bloodstream and improves circulation. It rejuvenates and is said to prolong life. It prepares the body for Pranayama.

## Comfortable Pranayama (Sukh Purvak)

This is an easier and less strenuous cleansing exercise.

Sit in one of the meditative postures. Close the right nostril with your right thumb. Inhale slowly and evenly through the left nostril, filling the lower (often neglected) parts of the lungs, then the middle and upper lungs. There must be no forcing. Retain the air for a few seconds, closing the left nostril with the left thumb. This breath suspension the Yogi calls kumbhaka. Then release the right nostril and exhale slowly through it.

Now repeat the process. Inhale through the right nostril, retain the air and exhale through the left nostril. This is one *round*.

The ratio favoured by experienced Yogis between inhalation, retention, and exhalation is 1:4:2. That is to say, if you inhale for five seconds, then suspend the breath for twenty seconds and exhale over a count of ten seconds. This is too severe a ratio for most Western students, who will be more comfortable with ratios of 1:1:1 or 1:1:2. The breath must always be even and kept under perfect control.

Perform five rounds.

### Benefits

Comfortable Pranayama aids digestion and improves the appetite. It cleanses the nasal passages and sinuses, and tones the nervous system. It also purifies and enriches the bloodstream and has a calming and concentrating effect on the mind.

## The Bellows Breath (Bhastrika)

This breathing exercise is so named because it imitates the action of a blacksmith's bellows.

In Bhastrika you inhale and exhale at the rate of about one inhalation and exhalation per second. As in Kapalabhati the inhalation should be twice as long as the exhalation, which is assisted by a quick instroke of the abdominal muscles and diaphragm. It differs from Kapalabhati in that a suspension of breath (kumbhaka) is added at the end of each round. There is also a variation using alternate instead of both nostrils.

Ten exhalations will be enough for one round at first but later you should be able to manage comfortably sixty exhalations in a round of one minute. At the completion of each round perform a kumbhaka as follows:

Inhale deeply and slowly through the right nostril (pingala) until the lungs are comfortably filled. Retain the breath for some seconds, then exhale slowly through the left nostril (ida). When all the air has been expelled inhale through the same nostril. Suspend again. Exhale through the right nostril.

This is done at the end of each round. When using one nostril the other is held closed with finger or thumb.

Yoga literature contains several slight variations of technique. Sometimes the kumbhaka is described with the use of both nostrils.

The chief variation is to use alternate instead of both nostrils in the 'bellows' part of Bhastrika. Close your left nostril. Exhale through the right nostril. Inhale through the same nostril and exhale sharply through the left nostril. This means releasing the left nostril and at the same time closing the right. Immediately you have expelled the air through the left nostril you inhale through it and exhale through the right nostril, and so on.

Perform three rounds. Take thirty seconds' rest, breathing freely between rounds.

### Benefits

The Bellows Breath energises, removes phlegm and cleanses the nasal passages and sinuses, purifies the bloodstream, aids digestion, prevents and cures disease, warms the body and tones the nervous system.

## *The Victorious Breath (Ujjayi)*

In Ujjayi you breathe through both nostrils. It differs from the other pranayamas in that the glottis remains half-closed during inhalation and exhalation. The glottis is the opening at the upper part of the windpipe and between the vocal cords which we contract and dilate in modulating our voices. This partial closure of the glottis produces a soft but clearly audible sound during breathing. The steadiness of this sound should be noted to see if the breathing is as smooth, slow and controlled as it should be.

Between inhalation and exhalation there is a suspension of breath which is assisted by the chin-lock (jalandhara). The chin is lowered and rested firmly in the jugular notch. On moderate breath suspension the use of the chin-lock is optional. The Yogis say that through breath retention, Prana can be sent to all parts of the body, 'from the nails of the toes to the tips of the hair.' Some of them develop the practice of breath suspension to such a degree that they can be buried for days without coming to any harm. We can marvel at, but need not try to emulate, such feats. Do not try to prolong breath suspension unduly. Besides the possibility of a strain of lungs or heart, if you suspend the breath over-long then exhalation will not be under full control. The air will be expelled violently or jerkily, instead of in the smooth, even manner required.

The Victorious Breath may be performed standing, and even when walking, as well as in the meditative postures. If performed during walking, the steps taken can be counted to provide the ratio between inhalation, suspension, and exhalation. People whose leisure time is limited should watch out for opportunities to practise Ujjayi in the course of their daily activities.

Perform five rounds. Rest for thirty seconds between rounds, breathing normally.

### Benefits

The Victorious Breath clears the nostrils and removes phlegm from the throat, tones the nervous system, purifies the bloodstream, aids digestion, improves health and vitality, and may be employed when courage is needed.

## The Hissing Sound Breath (Sitkari)

The nostrils and not the mouth are used for most Yogic breath controls, but in Sitkari air is taken in through the mouth and released through the nostrils. The lips are slightly parted and the tip of the tongue is pushed between the upper and lower sets of teeth. A little space is left between the tongue and the upper lip for air to be drawn in, producing a hissing sound. The breath is held for a few seconds, then exhaled through the nostrils.

Perform three rounds.

## Benefits

The Hissing Sound Breath cools the system, purifies the blood, appeases hunger and quenches thirst.

## *The Cooling Breath (Sitali)*

In the Cooling Breath the tongue is protruded between the lips and folded into a trough by curling up the outer edges. Air is drawn in slowly and smoothly along the folded tongue. The tongue is then drawn back into the mouth and the lips brought together for retention of air. Then the air is released smoothly through the *nostrils*.

Perform three rounds.

## Benefits

The benefits are as given for the Hissing Breath. In addition, the Cooling Breath is said to stimulate the liver and the spleen and to calm the nervous system.

These are the most important exercises of Pranayama. If Pranayama is performed carefully and as instructed, there will be an immediate increase in bodily vitality, and a tranquillising effect on the mind will be produced. But forcing or long breath suspensions must be avoided.

The *Hatha Yoga Pradipika* says:

> The air should be expelled with proper tact, and should be filled in skilfully, and should be kept confined properly. Thus it brings success. When the nadis (nerve channels) become free from impurities, and there appear the outward signs of success, such as lean body and glowing colour, then one should feel certain of success. By removing the impurities of the nadis the air can be restrained, according to one's wish, and the appetite is increased, the divine sound is awakened, and the body becomes healthy.

Breath control is at the very heart of Hatha Yoga practice. Here again we can see the sun (ha) and moon (tha) symbolism that is implicit in the name of this form of Yoga. The air passing through the right nostril is called the 'sun breath' and that passing through the left nostril is called the 'moon breath'. Hatha Yoga unifies the positive and negative, male and female, sun and moon energies.

Many books on Yoga concentrate on the postures and give scant attention to the breathing exercises. The breath controls are as important as the postures – perhaps more important. As we have seen, Hatha Yoga takes its name from the practice of Pranayama. A full account of Yogic breathing is given in *The Complete Yoga Book* (Rider).

# 7
# YOGA HYGIENE AND DIET

## —— The six purification practices ——

Yogis are very thorough in the matter of personal hygiene and many centuries ago they developed certain practices to remove impurities from the body. These show a singular understanding and control of the human body.

The six main cleansing acts (shat karmas) of Hatha Yoga are, giving their Sanskrit titles: Kapalabhati, Nauli, Basti, Dhauti, Neti and Trataka. Kapalabhati is a breathing exercise which cleanses the respiratory passages and the lungs, as described in Chapter 6 on 'Yoga Breathing'. Nauli is a muscle control in which the rectus abdominis, a pair of muscles in the centre of the abdomen, are isolated after exhaling fully and making a 'hollow tank' of the abdomen by allowing it to draw in towards the backbone. The Abdominal Retraction that precedes the performance of Nauli has the Sanskrit name Uddiyana; it is usually listed as a bandha or muscle lock, but the present chapter seems the appropriate place to describe its performance. Nauli has a key role in the practice of Basti, in which the Yogi squats in water and irrigates the colon by dilating the muscles of the anus. Dhauti, Neti, and Trataka are ways of cleansing the stomach, the nostrils, and the eyes respectively.

It is necessary to warn the student that the practice of Dhauti, Basti, and Neti in their traditional forms are not without hazards to health, unless practised under the supervision of a highly qualified teacher. Safer adaptations are possible in some cases. These will be indicated.

## *Abdominal retraction*

The muscle controls Uddiyani and Nauli should only be performed on an empty stomach. Empty the bladder, and the bowels also, if you can, before practice. Attempts to do these exercises on a full stomach will not be successful in creating a deep hollow, and there is danger of causing a hernia of the diaphragm. It is also essential to empty the lungs of air.

The best starting posture for learning these abdominal controls is to stand firmly with the legs about thirty centimetres apart, the knees slightly bent, the palm of the right hand on the right thigh and the palm of the left hand on the left thigh. The fingers are spread apart. Later, it

**Fig. 32   Abdominal retraction**

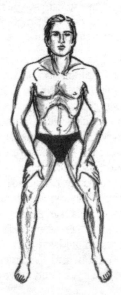

becomes easy to perform the controls in other postures – sitting in the Thunderbolt Posture is excellent for performing them – but nothing beats the standing posture described above for learning purposes. It also helps the beginner if he practises before a mirror and keeps his gaze on the centre of the abdomen as reflected in the glass.

Exhale, emptying the lungs, through both nostrils and mouth. Do this in two rapid rushes of air, with the briefest possible pause between. Without breathing in, expand and slightly raise the ribs, and draw back the abdomen towards the backbone, creating, as one old Hatha Yoga textbook puts it, 'a hollow tank'; the diaphragm rises into the cavity of the rib cage. With practice the control becomes easier and the retraction deeper – if you keep the abdominal wall relaxed, it will draw backwards and upwards as though being pulled involuntarily by a string attached to the backbone.

Hold the retraction a second, then release it and immediately retract again. The hollowing of the abdomen is repeated several times to each emptying of the lungs. As the muscles become stronger and more accustomed to the exercise, you should be able to perform ten to twenty quick retractions to one exhalation. This is called a *round*, and a rest of about fifteen seconds, breathing freely, should be taken before starting another round. Three rounds will be sufficient for most students, though the more experienced practitioner may perform four or five rounds.

Another way of exercising the abdomen through retraction, which may be alternated with the above method, is to exhale fully and then retract as before, holding the deep retraction for between five and ten seconds, before releasing. Whereas in the preceding method you perform ten to twenty quick retractions to one exhalation, you may now perform five to ten retractions that are each done separately. Take a pause of from five to ten seconds between each retraction. Then rest, breathing freely for one minute, before performing another round.

## Isolation of the recti muscles

The recti are a pair of muscles running from chest to pubis down the centre of the abdomen. While the remainder of the abdomen is retracted and remains passive, the recti may be brought forward in a somewhat

## Fig. 33　Isolation of the Recti Muscles

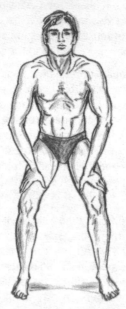

spectacular isolation. Success comes from performing Uddiyani with the abdomen relaxed, as described above. Pressing down with the hands on the thighs helps the beginner, as does fixing the gaze on the centre of the abdomen, reflected in a mirror. Avoid straining; the control takes some time to master, and is only possible when proficiency has been achieved in the first part, the abdominal retraction. The recti sit out in a thin wedge between ribcage and pelvis, with the abdomen on right and left deeply recessed. The breath must stay out and the lungs kept empty during the isolation.

The two methods of performance described for the retractions apply also to the isolations. In the first method, you hold each isolation for only one second and perform five to eight isolations on the one exhalation. Rest about a minute, breathing freely, then perform a second round of five to eight isolations. In the second method, one isolation only is performed to each exhalation, but it is sustained for five to ten seconds, according to comfort. This is a round. Rest, breathing freely, for about a minute, then perform a second round.

Once proficient in isolating the two recti, a further development in control is to isolate each separately. By alternately relaxing and contracting the right and left recti the abdominal muscles may be rolled from side to side in a wave-like motion, first in one direction, then the other.

The techniques of Abdominal Retractions and Isolation of the Recti Muscles are worth mastering. Do not worry if the isolations do not come easily to you. Concentrate on performing the deep retractions correctly and the control of the recti will come later.

### Benefits

These remarkable muscle controls are a key to defeating abdominal sag and spread. The abdominal wall and the important organs behind receive a massage that is both invigorating and rejuvenating. Surplus fat is removed. Metabolism, circulation, and digestion are improved. Natural, easy and regular bowel action is stimulated.

## *Cleansing the colon*

Isolation of the Recti Muscles (Nauli), as described above, plays an important part in the practise of Basti or irrigating the colon, performed by squatting in water and creating a vacuum in the lower bowel and so drawing up water. Success requires the ability to dilate and contract the circular muscles around the anus.

Teachers of Hatha Yoga and writers on Yoga are divided over whether there is or is not a need to irrigate the colon: some say it has great value to health, others say it is not necessary if the student follows a predominantly sattvic (pure) diet and practices the breath controls (pranayama) and the postures (asanas).

The method is as follows: The Yogi squats, chest against knees, in water that has been boiled and allowed to cool to luke-warm. The Yogi hollows the abdomen – on empty stomach, bladder, and bowels – and follows with Isolation of the Recti Abdominis, as instructed above. This creates a vacuum in the lower bowel. Water is drawn in if the circular muscles around the anus are dilated, and penetrates the colon, which is the greater part of the large intestine, ending in the rectum. About a litre of water may be taken into the colon. The water is retained a few minutes and then expelled in small amounts through control of the rectal muscles. The abdominal controls are continued during retention of the water in the colon, increasing the normal peristaltic action – the wavelike muscular contractions within the lining of the intestines. This helps water reach every part of the colon.

Yogis say that Basti is superior to the use of the modern enema. A greased enema nozzle may be inserted into the rectum by persons who have not yet mastered the control of the sphincters of the anus.

Penetration by water into the colon sometimes occurs spontaneously in swimmers whose abdomen is expanding and retracting vigorously following a race.

Some Yogis can draw water through the urethra, cleansing the bladder – a more difficult control than washing the colon.

## Cleansing the stomach

In the practice of Dhauti a long strip of cloth – surgical gauze three to four inches wide will do – is swallowed and allowed to rest in the stomach for some time before pulling it out. The cloth may be soaked in warm water or milk before being 'eaten' bit by bit. Swallowing only two or three feet at first, it is possible when the lining of the throat becomes accustomed to the practice to take in fifteen feet or more. At first there is an impulse to retch, but this passes. Several weeks of practice may be necessary before success is achieved. The cloth is allowed to remain in the stomach for ten to fifteen minutes before being pulled out slowly. If it remains longer than twenty minutes in the stomach, it will start passing through the intestines.

Dhauti removes phlegm, bile, and other impurities from the stomach, and is said to be helpful in curing some diseases.

An alternative method of cleansing the stomach is to drink several glasses of warm water in which salt has been dissolved until vomiting empties the stomach. This is called yamana dhauti.

Though Dhauti is still practised at some schools of Hatha Yoga in India, it cannot be recommended for experimentation by any student without an experienced teacher being present.

## Cleansing the nostrils

Neti is nasal cleansing. Traditionally, a soft cord is used, but the modern method is to use a catheter. The cord or catheter is passed through one nostril and out of the mouth and then drawn back and forth for a time before the process is repeated through the other nostril.

In the above method there is a risk of damaging or irritating the sensitive mucous membrane of the nostrils. A safer, alternative method is to sniff water through the nostrils and expel it from the mouth. This is called vyut-krama. It is possible to reverse this process and take the water through the mouth and expel it through the nostrils. This is sit-krama.

Boil a pint of water, then allow it to cool to about blood temperature. Add a teaspoonful of sea salt. Use a cup, bowl, or cupped hand to raise the water to the nostrils, leaving the mouth free. Sniff or draw the water up the nostrils in slow stages until it can be expelled from the mouth. Continue until the pint of water has been used. Then blow the nose thoroughly using clean tissues. After initial discomfort, one becomes used to the sensation of water in the nostrils.

Yogis say that regular nasal cleaning prevents colds, catarrh, sinusitis, and infections of the throat.

## Cleansing the eyes

Trataka consists of gazing steadily at a candle flame or any other mildly bright object, placed level with the eyes and a few feet before them. The Yogi continues gazing until the eyes begin to tire and to water. He then ends the exercise and washes the eyes with cold water. The Sanskrit source books claim that Trataka strengthens the eyes, may induce clairvoyance, and, as one of them puts it, 'should be kept secret very carefully, like a box of jewellery.'

When Trataka is performed as a meditation rather than as a hygiene, the eyes are closed after gazing for a few minutes at a candle flame, a coloured fifteen-watt bulb, or some other bright object: the after-image of the flame or object is then gazed upon with the mind's eye.

# ───── Oral hygiene ─────

As well as performing the six cleansing exercises, the Yogi gives attention to the cleanliness of his mouth. He rinses his mouth with water and cleans the root of his tongue and his gums by massaging them with the tips of the first and second fingers of one hand. He may also use the back of a spoon to scrape the tongue gently in an outward direction.

The teeth should be brushed regularly to keep them clear of tartar and bacterial plaque. Also have your teeth looked at by a dentist every six months.

# ───── Diet ─────

It should be obvious that if you are not to jeopardise the vitality that Yoga promotes you must give attention both to how and to what you eat.

Here, moderation is the rule. The Yogi is advised at a main meal to fill half of his stomach with food, one quarter with water, and keep one quarter empty. What this means is that at any meal you should eat enough to satisfy your hunger, but not so much as to give a gorged feeling.

The foods recommended by the classic Yoga texts include many that have no meaning to the average Westerner – mudga and masa beans, jack-fruit, jujubes, bonduc nuts, patola leaves, and so on. Others 'very beneficial to those who practise Yoga' are available to all: wheat, rice, barley, corn, wheaten bread, milk, honey and fresh vegetables.

A lacto-vegetarian diet is favoured by Yoga – that is, a diet based on vegetables and milk and milk products. However, abstinence from fish and meat is not insisted upon by many gurus, especially those teaching Westerners.

For a long time vegetarianism was severely criticised by the Western medical profession on the grounds that such a diet missed out on vital nutrients. Today, the profession, in the main, grants that a well-planned vegetarian diet will supply the body's needs for fuel to supply energy and to repair tissues; it is now also generally recognised that adequate protein, which does the work of repair and renewal, can be obtained from vegetable sources, such as soya beans and whole cereals, and from milk and cheese. This is the basis of the Yoga diet.

The instructions on diet given in the classic texts of Hatha Yoga are useful only as guidelines for today, however, certain unchanging principles have guided Yoga's attitude to diet through the centuries.

Yoga masters recommend a diet of sattvic or 'pure' foods, and warn against rajasic or stimulating food and tamasic or impure food. Sattvic foods are milk, milk products, fruits, vegetables and grains.

This is the basis of a lacto-vegetarian diet of the kind followed by most leading teachers of Yoga and expected of students joining an ashram or Yoga school.

It is noticeable that most of the sattvic foods are alkaline-forming, neutralising acids in the body. Most Westerners eat too many acid-forming foods – meats, eggs, sugars, and starches principally – causing acidosis, whose symptoms are lassitude, headaches, nausea, insomnia and poor appetite.

Most Yogis are lacto-vegetarians principally because they link purity of diet with spiritual development, seeing a correlation between the quality and nature of the foods men eat and the quality of their spiritual life. But just as they believe that eating certain types of food may assist purification of the spiritual life so, too, they believe that the regular practice of Yoga postures, breathing exercises, and meditation leads to a modification of the diet and of eating habits. The Yogic approach is one of moderation in all things, and faddism has no place in it. It does seem to be the case that Yoga practice tends to lead the practitioner naturally to a decrease in desire for meat and to be more attracted by a diet of fruits, greens, whole cereals, milk and dairy products, with a corresponding aversion to refined, processed, and tinned foods.

## Some simple guidelines

Sound nutrition builds a wall of protection against stress and the degenerative diseases. The following dietary guidelines are recommended to readers who wish to eat for health and to obtain optimum results from their Yoga practice.

## (a) Become acquainted with the salient factors in sound nutrition.

Your health – perhaps even life itself – could depend on your having such knowledge. Briefly, what is required is a balanced supply of the six nutrients: proteins, fats, carbohydrates, water, vitamins, and mineral salts.

*Proteins* provide energy, but their special value is for repair and growth of tissues. Animal food proteins can be obtained from meat, poultry, eggs, milk and cheese, and plant proteins from whole grains, nuts, seeds and pulses (peas, beans, and lentils). Fish meat is one of the most concentrated and economical sources of protein – and it is more easily digested than animal meat.

*Fats* are a very rich energy source, but it is important to note that a high intake of animal fats has been linked by researchers with narrowing of the arteries, high blood pressure and heart attacks.

The main role of the *Carbohydrates* – mostly sugars and starches – is to supply fuel for combustion and energy. Whole grain foods are a healthy source. Refined sugar has little left of the nutrients naturally present in the sugar cane or sugar beet, but natural sugars are present in fresh and dried fruits, vegetables, milk – and some other foods.

*Water* has a vital role in the functioning of the human body and makes up about 70 per cent of bodyweight. Each person excretes more than two litres of moisture each day, which has to be replaced. An insufficient intake of water may cause constipation and endanger the health of the kidneys and the liver. It makes sense to drink a variety of beverages. Fruit and vegetable juices are rich in vitamins and mineral salts.

## (b) Recognise the importance of fibre in your diet.

Fibre (plant cellulose) is not of nutritional importance in itself, but it adds bulk to food passing through the intestinal tract, keeping it moist and on the move, and so promoting regular and efficient elimination of waste.

The best sources of fibre are grains, vegetables and fruits. You will probably benefit from taking a tablespoonful or two daily of wheat bran, the protective outer coating of the whole grain, taken as a supplement. It is most often taken with a breakfast cereal, though it may also be sprinkled on yoghourt, soups and some other foods.

## (c) Favour the alkaline-forming foods.

As mentioned above, the traditional Yoga diet favours alkaline-forming foods. Our blood is naturally slightly alkaline, and the body has ways of maintaining the alkaline-acid balance – such as calling on alkaline reserves and expelling excess acid in the urine. We can, however, help the body stay healthy and the mind and nervous system calm by ensuring that we eat plenty of alkaline-forming foods every day. Most Westerners are hooked on a diet that is predominantly acid-forming. The main acid-forming foods are meat, poultry, fish, eggs, cheese and the grains that compose the breakfast cereal, bread, etc. Yoga's traditional lacto-vegetarian diet is predominantly alkaline-forming. Whole and skimmed milk are alkaline, and most vegetables and fruits; even the citrus fruits that taste acid in the mouth make an alkaline contribution to the blood. So eat fruits and vegetables once or twice every day.

## (d) Base your diet on wholefoods.

Refining foods robs them of important nutrients, and while most of the several thousand chemicals used in food manufacturing may be safe, a question mark hangs over many of them. Reading the labels on foods in your supermarket is a wise precaution, avoiding those with a large amount of listed 'E' numbers. The inclusion of wholefoods in the daily diet ensures a good supply of nutrients and fibre. Let whole grains make the main contribution to your breakfast. Wholemeal bread contains the enzymes and vitamins E and B complex found in the whole grain. It is healthful to eat some raw vegetables and fruits daily. Fresh fruits are enjoyable to eat and most are alkaline-forming. Most raw vegetables are also alkaline-forming and supply the minerals magnesium and potassium, which help relax muscles, nervous system, and mind; in this they are allies of Yoga practice. Wash vegetables and fruits thoroughly. Pulses, seeds and grains are easily sprouted and their sprouts make a useful contribution to the diet. All you have to do is soak them overnight, rinse them three times a day thereafter, and succulent sprouts are ready for eating in three to five days. Empty out the water used for overnight soaking and rinse in clean water three times a day. Cooking depletes foods of some of their vitamin and mineral content, so cook vegetables as lightly as possible. In discussing Yoga's lacto-vegetarian diet, we should remember that the milk referred to in the classical Yoga texts was, of course, unpasturised. Pasturisation is another of those modern processes which, for whatever reason, take away from the natural properties of whole foods. Pasturisation alters the structure of the amino acid caseinogen in milk, and at the same time coagulates the calcium content. Pasturised milk is less easily digested than unpasturised milk and many people are allergic to it.

## (e) Seek balance and variety in your diet.

Balance and moderation are good rules for all aspects of living, and especially in diet. Whatever the merits of a single food, drink or dietary supplement, it should have only a balanced place in the total diet. This applies as much to so-called 'health foods' as to conventional foods. (A few years ago a man in England turned yellow and died from drinking excessive quantities of carrot juice!) Unless you are the victim of food allergies, beware of diets based on a restricted list of foods. Remember that a diet containing a wide variety of wholesome foods offers a balanced supply of nutrients – and our taste buds welcome it too.

The rule about variety extends to beverages as well as to foods. That way you avoid any dangers to health that might result from drinking too much of one particular beverage.

## (f) Cultivate 'body wisdom'.

The practitioner of Yoga develops 'body wisdom' – that is, awareness of how the body reacts to work and to play, to exercise and to rest. This awareness, with sensitive application, extends to knowing when your body wants or does not want food, how much to be taken comfortably at each meal, and eventually how your body reacts to particular foods. This awareness is particularly helpful for people who are allergic to certain (often common) foods. Allergy foods can be spotted by eliminating foods from the diet for several days and then reintroducing them; if you are allergic to them your body will let you know in some way.

A preference for wholefoods as opposed to refined foods grows with developing body wisdom. However, cravings for sugar, salt and stimulants may have to be overcome for body wisdom to be free to develop.

## (g) Break your addictions.

Food manufacturers know that millions of people are 'hooked' on sugary foods and sweeten their foods to boost profits. Sweets, chocolate, cakes, spoonfuls of sugar in tea and coffee, can give quick energy 'shots'. The trouble is that though the sugar goes quickly into the bloodstream, a fatigue rebound occurs in two or three hours, and the sugar addict is left craving another 'fix'. Many people suffer a rebound from their energy peaks that takes their blood below a healthy sugar level – the condition called hypoglycaemia. Paradoxically, people with a 'sweet tooth' are prone to low blood sugar. Breaking an addiction to sugar requires determination and holding in mind the benefits that result from overcoming the habit.

Another common addiction is to salt. Salt was once valuable as a preservative, but in these days of widespread ownership of fridges and freezers it is easy to supply the body with enough sodium (salt) from meat, vegetables and fruit. Researchers have linked high salt consumption with high blood pressure. And salt provides the same kind of stimulation as caffeine (in tea and coffee). It activates the adrenal glands which produce the hormones released in stressful situations.

## (h) Be aware of the dangers from saturated fats.

Cholesterol and other products in saturated animal fats have been linked with high blood pressure and heart disease. Wise precautions are to eat lean rather than fatty meats, and skimmed or semi-skimmed milk rather than whole milk. There has been widespread publicity favouring margarines high in polyunsaturated fatty acids; they are said to be less of a danger to the heart than butter. Unfortunately, recent research indicates that the hydrogenation of vegetable fats – i.e. passing hydrogen through them – cause the flat molecules of vegetable fats to stick together like wet plates, whereas butter's spherical molecules easily separate when digested. Butter, it would seem, is actually less threatening to the arteries than hydrogenated margarines, though a moderate use is indicated.

The saturated fats and cholesterol investigation is not without controversy. Some researchers have found that the dangers from dietary fat and cholesterol may be negated by a cheerful and relaxed attitude to life. Whether this is so or not, such an attitude is worth cultivating for other reasons, such as lowering tension and improving relationships with others.

## (i) Do not overeat.

Give your digestive processes a chance to do their work efficiently. When having a meal, leave a quarter of your stomach free, as old Yoga texts advise. A meal should be of sufficient bulk to satisfy hunger, but should not overtax the digestive or eliminative organs, thereby taking blood away from the brain and causing fuzzy consciousness. Masticating thoroughly prevents overeating.

Overeating is the principal cause of obesity. The overweight are prone to many complaints and diseases: diseases of the liver, kidneys and heart, diabetes, gout, high blood pressure and digestive disorders.

Eating for health and a high-fibre diet will help normalise figure and body weight; dietary control should be accompanied by the practice of Yoga postures and breath controls.

## (j) Consider taking a daily vitamin and mineral supplement.

Ideally, your diet should be so complete that you obtain all the vitamins and minerals needed for optimum health. But many people feel that this goal is not easy to attain and support their diet with a daily vitamin and mineral supplement. Numerous studies have shown that a lack of this or that vitamin leads to a certain illness or behaviour problem, and an experiment carried out in 1987 in Britain with schoolchildren showed that those given a daily vitamin and mineral supplement soon showed improvement in non-verbal intelligence.

## (k) Chew your food thoroughly.

Yogis attach great importance to this. Solid foods should be broken down and reduced to a liquid before passing into the stomach. This initial breaking down takes place in the mouth through chewing and the action of the saliva. Mastication is a necessary part of the digestive processes and should not be hurried or neglected.

## (l) Do not eat when excited or emotionally upset.

Emotional excitement impedes the flow of gastric juices in the stomach, resulting in indigestion. Many of the postures of Yoga aid digestion and prevent indigestion.

## (m) Enjoy what you eat.

Eating for health and eating for pleasure can go together. A healthy diet is not a punishing or ascetic choice of foods. If the broad outline of your approach to diet is healthy, then there is no need to become obsessive or fanatical about food. And there can be times, body allowing, when you can be flexible. Cultivate skill in preparing and cooking foods for health. Books on wholefood cookery will prove a good investment both in terms of encouraging a nutritious diet and enjoying it.

# 8

# MAKING THE MOST OF THE EXERCISES

The advice given here will help you to plan a basic Yoga programme, based on the postures already described. Detailed descriptions of these basic programmes are summarised at the end of the chapter for quick reference.

## —— How much time is needed? ——

You will naturally be wondering how much time you need devote to Yoga exercises to benefit from them. Any time given to them will not be wasted, but for satisfactory results fifteen to thirty minutes daily should be devoted to the postures and breath controls combined. Beginners should start with the basic programme taking fifteen minutes.

After two months of regular practice, add the Standing Forward Bend Posture and the Headstand and take twenty minutes. The programmes with a suggested length of ten minutes and five minutes are only intended for use on those occasions when circumstances do not allow a full programme. The basic programme may be built upon by the addition of advance postures, but do not practise for more than thirty minutes.

One hears the protest again and again: 'I would like to have more vitality, better health, a more youthful appearance, a tranquil mind . . . but I haven't the time to spare for exercises.' But is there a person living – no matter how full his daily activities – who could not find time (and lots of it) for some worthwhile task?

Try this experiment. For one whole day, from rising in the morning to retiring to bed in the evening, write down how you spent your time. At the end of the day you will be amazed to find the number of minutes – probably hours – that have been occupied by nothing of importance. This is true even for those people who claim they never have a minute to spare. If you utilise this time and add to it an extra half-hour a day through rising that much earlier in the morning, you will, believe it or not, be 'making' several weeks' extra time per year. Work it out for yourself.

This book has been written in the knowledge that most of its readers will be busy people – but the time required daily for the practice of Yoga can easily be 'made', as has just been shown, and it is surely worth using it in order to gain greater physical health and tranquility of mind.

## Time and place

Your daily Yoga practice may take place at any time you wish provided at least two hours have elapsed following a meal. A regular time each day should be fixed. Usually the most suitable times are in the morning on rising, late afternoon, or shortly before retiring to bed in the evening. Morning exercises give a good start to the day, though not everyone is at their most flexible at that time. Postures may be performed in the morning and meditation in the evening; but the arrangement may just as easily be reversed.

Wash yourself all over with cold or luke-warm water, followed by brisk towelling so that the skin is clean and glowing.

Follow this by brushing your teeth and rinsing your mouth with water. Wet the first and second fingers of one hand and massage the gums and the tongue with them. Rinse out your mouth with two or three cupfuls of water.

Place a folded blanket or a rug on the floor of a well-aired, but not cold or draughty, room. You may, of course, wish to exercise outdoors if the weather is suitable. Wear as little clothing as possible; what is worn should be loose-fitting. Women find that leotards provide comfort and freedom of movement.

# ___ A basic programme of postures ___ taking 15 minutes

The following programme of postures takes only fifteen minutes to complete and provides a balanced sequence for beginners and for all students requiring a basic programme which can be expanded and developed as strength and suppleness increase. The more advanced postures may be added gradually as they are mastered. The postures have been chosen to exercise the whole body from head to toe. As pointed out earlier (on page 34), back bends tend to exaggerate any distortions in the spine. Group forward bends are earlier in your programme, for they will straighten the vertebral column and correctly align it. Backwards bends always follow forward bends. Similarly, the Headstand (if practised) should precede performance of the Shoulder-stand or Plough Postures.

Each posture should be held steadily for the target time, or as near to it as can be sustained comfortably. In most cases the target time is one minute.

The right mental attitude contributes to the efficacy of the programme. It is in the essential spirit of Yoga to give your full attention and awareness to each moment of the programme – going into a posture, staying in it, and coming out of it. In the rest pauses between postures you should close your eyes and detach yourself from whatever is going on around you. Ten seconds may seem a short period of rest, but it is of great value if there is a full 'letting go' in the Yogic manner.

## 1 The Spinal Rock – Target time: 1 minute

Limber-up with the Spinal Rock (see p. 34). Make sure you have a
blanket or some other soft layer beneath the spine – a hard surface could
be painful for the spine and perhaps do some damage. Roll yourself into a
'ball', keeping your knees together and hugging the thighs, which are
against the chest. Rock backwards and forwards for one minute. Remember to breathe in as you go forwards and breathe out as you rock
backwards.

Stretch out flat on your back, the legs fully extended, and rest, really
'letting go' and with your eyes closed, for ten seconds.

## 2 The Tree Posture – Target time: 30 seconds on each foot

Stand up and give your body a full-length stretch with the Tree Posture
(see p. 35), which also tones the body and improves poise. It strengthens
the muscles that work to hold the body erect on its middle line, a line
visible down the centre of the trunk and abdomen and of the back in
Greek statues and in athletic figures today. It makes an excellent opening
posture. Balance first on the left foot and then on the right foot, holding
the body as straight and upright as possible, for up to thirty seconds for
each foot. Through time the posture will be held with greater steadiness
– a sign of increasing stability in the nervous system. Remember that
balance is helped by fixing the gaze on a point directly in front of you at
eye-level.

## 3 The Back-Stretching Posture – Target time: 30 seconds. Perform twice

Staying on your back with the legs fully extended and together, raise
your head and trunk into a sitting position in readiness for the Back-
stretching Posture (see p. 40). Breathe out, and stretch forward and
down, without moving your legs. Even if your forward stretch does not
enable you to grasp your feet or to lower your face on to your knees, your
comfortable limit of stretching will be doing you as much good as that

gained by the more supple student. Hold your ankles if you cannot grasp your feet. Hold the fully stretched position for up to thirty seconds. Perform again.

Later you will be able to add the Knee and Head Posture (see p. 61) in which only one leg is extended and you lower the upper body down on it.

Return unhurriedly to lying flat on your back and rest in that position for ten seconds.

## 4  The Shoulderstand Posture – Target time: 1 minute

Now lie flat on your back on the floor and rest totally for ten seconds. Then, supporting the lower back with the palms of the hands, raise the legs and the trunk slowly to a straight vertical position, until the body is supported only by the shoulders and the upper arms. The Shoulderstand (see p. 45) is well named the 'all body' posture, for all the body is involved in the position and benefits from it. For a great many people the Yoga Headstand is too severe – but the Shoulderstand provides a satisfactory substitute.

The Shoulderstand Posture is one of the most popular classic poses of Hatha Yoga. Breathe freely, using the abdominal muscles, and hold the pose perfectly straight and unwavering for up to one minute. Remember that the elbows should not be spaced more widely apart than the width of the shoulders, and to keep the legs and feet relaxed. It is not a suitable posture for persons with stiff or arthritic necks.

In the Half-Shoulderstand Posture, which is for people who cannot manage the full Shoulderstand Posture, the legs and the trunk form an angle and the hands support the hips rather than the lower back.

In the Balancing Shoulderstand Posture, which is for advanced students, the support of the hands is removed and the arms are fully extended along the floor in line with the shoulders and at shoulders' width, or placed horizontally alongside the body.

It is important to come out of this and other postures slowly. It is against the spirit of Yoga to make hurried or jerky movements. Lower your back slowly to the floor, keeping the legs upright, at an angle of ninety degrees to the floor. Then slowly lower the legs to the floor.

Rest flat on your back for ten seconds.

## 5 The Plough Posture – Target time: 1 minute

Again raise your legs and trunk to a perpendicular position, supporting the body on the upper arms and the shoulders with the palms of the hands against the lower back. But this time make the Shoulderstand Posture the starting position for the Plough Posture (see p. 50), which removes tension and stiffness from the spine. The legs are kept straight and are lowered until the toes touch the floor behind your head. In expert performance the feet drop slowly of their own weight until the toes rest on the floor.

Don't be put off by initial failures, for spinal suppleness improves rapidly if you practise daily. Lower the legs as far as you can. Hold the final position for up to one minute. Breathe freely.

Unwind slowly by going into the Shoulderstand Posture and then coming down in the manner indicated for that posture above. Lying flat on your back, rest for ten seconds.

## 6 The Cobra Posture – Target time: 30 seconds. Perform twice

Turn over and lie face down, your forehead resting on the floor, in preparation for the Cobra Posture (see p. 51). Bend the arms and place the palms of the hands on the floor, level with and close to the shoulders, the fingers pointing straight forward. The legs are fully extended with the knees and the ankles touching. Slowly raise the head and then the shoulders and the upper back. Feel each vertebra bend. Hold the final position for up to thirty seconds. Feel each vertebra unwind as you slowly return the upper body to the floor.

Turn on to your back with the legs fully extended together. Rest, letting go fully, for ten seconds. Perform again.

## 7 The Bow Posture – Target time: 30 seconds. Perform twice

Turn over and lie face down on the floor for the Bow Posture (see p. 53) which bends the spine in the opposite direction to that required for the preceding Back-stretching Posture. This is not an easy posture to perform as effectively as one usually sees it depicted in book illustrations: at first the thighs tend to refuse to lift up from the floor. Practice brings increasing success. It will be easier to form a 'bow' if at first the legs are kept a little apart and gradually brought closer together as the body becomes stronger and more supple. Sustain the curved position for up to thirty seconds. Perform again.

Release the 'drawn bow' and lie motionless for ten seconds.

## 8 The Mountain Posture – Target time: 1 minute

The sitting Mountain Posture (see p. 58), when compared with the Bow Posture, is simple and almost effortless, though highly beneficial in many ways. The final position has a stable restfulness that is made more enjoyable by the contrast with the preceding positions that exercised the spine.

Sit in any of the cross-legged positions described on pages 78–80. You may sit on a chair if you are uncomfortable when sitting cross-legged. The palms of the hands are brought together overhead, with the fingers pointing directly upwards. Stretch the arms up, keeping the back upright and the chin level. Breathe deeply into the abdomen and look straight ahead. Stay immobile for up to one minute. In the Mountain Posture there is an immediate feeling of calmness and strength.

Now adopt the Thunderbolt Posture (see p. 54), sitting on the heels with the knees together and the big toes touching. Keep the back straight and the head and back in a vertical, erect line. Sit motionless for ten seconds.

The Thunderbolt Posture provides the basic position for performance of postures nine and ten in this programme.

## 9 The Lion Posture – Target time: 30 seconds. Perform twice

The Lion Posture (see p. 56) does not provide the prettiest of sights, but it exercises a set of muscles that are usually neglected. Most exercise systems work the muscles between the neck and the feet, and miss out the muscles of the face, which, if you think about it, are the most important set of muscles human beings possess. They are the muscles most exposed to the gaze of other people, and on which our character is judged. They provide a subtle interplay of expression in response to the shifting nuances of our emotional life.

What is so often overlooked is that the muscles of the face respond to exercise in exactly the same way as do the arms or the legs or the muscles of the trunk. That is to say, the facial muscles when exercised regularly are strengthened, toned, and firmed, taking on more youthful and attractive contours. I was surprised when press, radio, and television responded with interest to publication of *New Faces* (Thorsons) on the grounds that here was a surprising and novel idea. To my mind what is surprising is that people who are keen to make their bodies as youthful and healthful as possible stop exercising at the neck.

The Lion Posture brings all the facial muscles into action in a static (isometric) contraction that flushes the face with blood and counteracts weakening and sagging of the facial muscles. A contraction lasting only ten seconds leaves the face glowing and animated. Sit quietly for ten seconds, then repeat the facial and bodily contraction, again for ten seconds.

Take another rest lasting ten seconds.

The facial tissues also benefit from the flow of blood into them during the inverted postures of Yoga, such as the Shoulderstand and the Headstand, and the neck and the jawline are firmed and shaped by the Bow, the Cobra, and many other postures.

## The clock

This is another Yoga exercise with a bearing on how our faces feel to ourselves and look to others. Sit cross-legged, on the heels in the

Thunderbolt Posture, or on a chair. Keep the back straight and the head level. Moving only the eyes, look up as though to the figure twelve on an imaginary clock, then almost immediately down as though to six o'clock, and so on, right round the clock. Repeat, working in an anti-clockwise direction: twelve – six, eleven – five, ten – four, and so on. Conclude by circling the eyes a few times, first in a clockwise direction and then in an anti-clockwise direction. Other exercise systems tend to neglect the movements of the eyes, but exercise prevents eye fatigue and brightens the expression of the face. Most people do not move their eyes sufficiently often to maintain their mobility: they turn the head to look right or left and tilt the head to look up or down. One should sometimes move the eyes instead of the head and give them some exercise.

## 10 The Cowface Posture – Target time: thirty seconds to each side

The great value of the oddly named Cowface Posture (see p. 57) is the way it straightens and strengthens the back and improves posture. No student need miss out on it – even if you cannot make the fingers of the right and left hands lock, the exercise can still be performed beneficially by stretching a handkerchief or a towel tautly between the hands, shortening the gap as flexibility increases in the shoulder-joints. Eventually one day the fingertips will touch and shortly afterwards they may be locked together. The aid of a handkerchief or a towel will then no longer be necessary.

The Cowface posture should on no account be left out of a programme by persons following sedentary occupations in which they have to look down and bend forward. Indeed, people who spend several hours of a working day bending over a desk or a bench should several times a day sit up straight or stand up straight and squeeze the shoulderblade muscles together by linking fingers along the centre line of the back. The Cowface Posture takes tension out of the shoulders and the upper back. It strengthens the muscles that hold the shoulderblades together and straightens a rounded upper back.

Having linked fingers along the centre line of the back, while sitting upright in the Thunderbolt Posture, sustain the Cowface position for up to thirty seconds. Reverse the roles of the arms in the posture and repeat, again for up to thirty seconds.

## 11 The Relaxation Posture – Target time: 2 minutes minimum

You should conclude every programme of postures with the Relaxation or Corpse Posture (see p. 71), which rests, relaxes and prepares both body and mind for the return to varied activity. The mental attitude during Savasana is important for its success and can make even a couple of minutes' relaxation valuable, though if possible you should spend five minutes or more 'letting go' totally. The pose has to be learned mentally as well as physically. Correct body posture has to be matched by correct 'inner posture', a mental attitude of detaching the mind from what is going on round about.

Dr Pandit Shiv Sharma, who holds the highest title of the Indian medical profession, that of Vaidya Ratna, says of Savasana: 'This posture has been successfully utilised by eminent modern cardiologists in India to speed up the recovery of patients convalescing from heart diseases. It has been observed that patients practising Savasana recover more quickly and completely. It also acts as a prophylactic against heart diseases in general. Practice of this posture helps to prevent the harmful effects on the body and mind of undue stress or anxiety, whether physical or mental. If one can achieve the right amount of detachment while relaxing in this pose, the feeling of relaxation will be far superior to that experienced from the use of tranquillisers and sedatives.'

## The Standing Forward Bend Posture (see p. 39)

This may be added to the above programme by bringing it between the Tree Posture and the Shoulderstand Posture. A reviewer of the first edition of this book, for the *Times Educational Supplement*, expressed surprise that some Yogic postures show close similarities to exercises most Westerners learn as children, and likened the discovery to the surprise of M. Jourdain in Molière's *Le Bourgeois Gentilhomme*, who found he had been talking prose for forty years and had never known it. The reviewer had probably mostly in mind the Standing Forward Bend and its similarities to the 'toes touch' of Western calisthenics. The comparison is superficial. The Westerner performs the 'toes touch' quickly and bounces up immediately; the Yogi's performance is a slow stretch. The Westerner repeats the quick movement again and again until sweating and breathing fast; the Yogi folds the body as fully as possible and stays down for up to a minute, or more. In practice this exercise should be repeated once.

The Headstand (see p. 41) may also be incorporated in the above programme, if it is not too severe for you. It will fit in before the Shoulderstand Posture. Remember that it should not be practised by persons who suffer from high blood pressure, heart complaints, or diseases of the brain, eyes, and ears. Nor is it suitable for the older person taking up Yoga. The Shoulderstand makes an excellent substitute for the Headstand. And if even the Shoulderstand is too vigorous, lying at an angle with the feet raised higher than the head is refreshing. When Dad puts his stockinged or slippered feet on the mantelpiece, he may not know it, but he is making use of old Yogic wisdom about the body and the replenishment of its energies.

You should progress to the full Headstand by means of the Half-Headstand, without straightening the legs. When you feel confident in the Half-Headstand and can sustain it steadily for two minutes, you may then slowly straighten your legs into a vertical position and complete the full Headstand.

The two walls of a corner in a room may be used to give support in early practice. Don't rush matters. Beginners should practise the Half-Headstand for several weeks before doing the full Headstand. Then work up from two minutes in the Headstand to five minutes, adding more portions of a minute gradually over several weeks. Only increase the duration of the fully inverted position if you are comfortable and experience no dizziness or harmful side-effects. Five minutes will be a satisfactory limit for most students and only very experienced practitioners should exceed it.

## The abdominal controls

The abdominal muscle controls of Retraction (Uddiyana) and Isolation of the Recti (Nauli) have not been included in the basic programme because they may be practised on an empty stomach along with morning ablutions. An empty or nearly empty stomach and full exhalations are essential for success. Some weeks of daily practice of the Retractions are usually necessary before the Isolations are mastered.

Breathe out fully and perform one to twenty contractions, according to your ability. Take fifteen seconds' rest and then do another round. After three or four weeks add a third round.

## Sitting postures

The cross-legged sitting postures (see pp. 78–80) should be used for a few minutes daily, as opportunity presents, when reading, watching TV, and so on.

# ——————— Advanced postures ———————

The advanced postures are those that present most difficulty for the majority of people learning Yoga. A person's build – for example, the proportionate lengths of the arms, trunk, and legs – have a bearing on which poses are easy and which are difficult. So, in some cases, what have been called advanced postures in this book may be soon mastered. Similarly, a person's build may make some postures forever difficult. In many photographically illustrated books on Yoga, you will find that some postures have not been depicted, because they did not suit the model. Sometimes a second model is used for these postures.

Fortunately, most postures can be adapted or simplified. This is essential for most Western students, though the very supple Indian masters do not always allow for the lack of mobility in the joints of their Western students, who, for one thing, are not accustomed to sitting cross-legged on the ground after the years of childhood have passed.

The advanced postures may be added to the basic programme as suppleness permits. They are not essential to the obtaining of better health through Yoga, though many students master at least some of them. If dropping some postures from the basic programme to replace them with other postures, I would advise leaving in the Shoulderstand, the Plough, the Back-stretching Posture. These three postures are too important to leave out of a programme, unless briefly.

## The Yoga Cat Stretch

This is a combination of several postures and is useful when time is strictly limited. Yogis of old devised it after studying the stretching actions of the jungle cats. You will observe that similar movements are performed by the domestic cat.

Stand upright with the feet together, then lean forward and place the palms of your hands apart on the floor at shoulders' width. Breathe out and draw back the abdomen. The arms and the legs should be straight. Hold the buttocks as high as possible and support the body on the hands and the toes. Keep your chin tucked in against your chest so that you are gazing at your feet. This is the first position.

Bending your arms, bring your head and shoulders downwards and forwards in a sweeping, circular motion. The chest should sweep low and touch the floor as it passes between the hands. Breathing in, straighten

**Fig. 34   Cat Stretch**

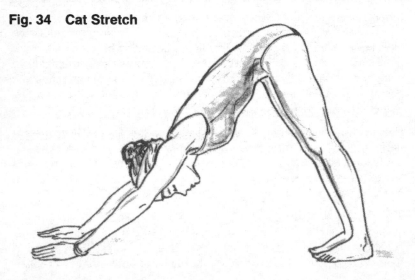

your arms. At the completion of the movement, which should be smooth and unhurried, the back will be arched and the chin tilted up, so that the eyes gaze at the ceiling. Use your arms to push the body upwards and backwards. You will recognise this second key position as identical to the Cobra Posture.

Hold the Cobra Posture for two or three seconds before returning to the first position, in which the hips are held high, by reversing the movement described. Breathe out as you return to the first position.

Perform five downward sweeps.

## The breathing exercises

The breath controls may be performed before or following the postures or at a separate time. Follow the instructions given in Chapter 6. They need only take five to ten minutes.

Start with either the Cleansing Breath (see p. 82) or the milder Comfortable Pranayana (see p. 83). After you have done either of these relax for fifteen seconds, breathing normally. Then commence the Bellows Breath (Bhastrika) (see p. 84). This can be done using both nostrils or alternate nostrils. When preceding it with the Cleansing Breath, I prefer the variation using alternate nostrils. If starting with the Comfortable Pranayama, use both nostrils for the Bellows Breath. Breathe normally for fifteen seconds, then complete the breathing exercises with the Victorious Breath (see p. 85). Remember that smooth control is needed throughout if the full benefits are to be received.

Add the Hissing Breath and the Cooling Breath in hot weather.

In all the breath controls have a mental picture of your body being flooded with the cosmic energy of Prana. Feel the Prana being carried on the enriched bloodstream to every cell in your body.

## Daily programmes

The programme of postures described earlier in this chapter should take about fifteen minutes, including the rest pauses, or twenty minutes if you add the Standing Forward Bend Posture and the Yoga Headstand Posture.

Summaries of some daily programmes, based on the basic Postures, are set out below with an indication of the number of minutes you should take to perform each posture. Advanced postures may be introduced at a later stage, building on the basic programme.

The suggested sequence of breathing exercises is also tabled.

If you want at any time to make the most of five minutes, perform the Cat Stretch and follow it with Comfortable Pranayama or the Cleansing Breath, giving two and a half minutes to each.

—— **15-minute basic programme** ——

| | **Postures** | **Minutes** |
|---|---|---|
| 1 | Spinal Rock | 1 |
| 2 | Tree Posture (Vrkasana) | 1 |
| | (*Perform to each side*) | |
| 3 | Back-stretching Posture (Paschimottanasana) | 1 |
| | (*Perform twice*) | |
| 4 | Shoulderstand Posture (Sarvangasana) | 1 |
| 5 | Plough Posture (Halasana) | 1 |
| 6 | Cobra Posture (Bhujangasana) | 1 |
| | (*Perform twice*) | |
| 7 | Bow Posture (Dhanurasana) | 1 |
| | (*Perform twice*) | |
| 8 | Mountain Posture (Parbatasana) | 1 |
| 9 | Lion Posture (Simhasana) | 1 |
| | (*Perform twice*) | |
| 10 | Cowface Posture (Gomukhasana) | 1 |
| | (*Perform to each side*) | |
| 11 | Relaxation Posture (Savasana) | 2 |
| | Rests and time taken going into and leaving postures | 3 |
| | TOTAL TIME | 15 |

## —— 20-minute basic programme ——

| | Postures | Minutes |
|---|---|---|
| 1 | Spinal Rock | 1 |
| 2 | Tree Posture (Vrkasana) | 1 |
| | (*Perform to each side*) | |
| 3 | Standing Forward Bend (Padahastasana) | 1 |
| 4 | Back-stretching Posture (Paschimottanasana) | 1 |
| | (*Perform twice*) | |
| 5 | Headstand Posture (Sirsasana) | 3 |
| 6 | Shoulderstand Posture (Sarvangasana) | 1 |
| 7 | Plough Posture (Halasana) | 1 |
| 8 | Cobra Posture (Bhujangasana) | 1 |
| 9 | Bow Posture (Dhanurasana) | 1 |
| | (*Perform twice*) | |
| 10 | Mountain Posture (Parbatasana) | 1 |
| 11 | Lion Posture (Simhasana) | 1 |
| | (*Perform twice*) | |
| 12 | Cowface Posture (Gomukhasana) | 1 |
| | (*Perform to each side*) | |
| 13 | Relaxation Posture (Savasana) | 2 |
| | Rests and time taken going into and leaving postures | 4 |
| | TOTAL TIME | 20 |

## —— 10-minute basic programme ——

| | Postures | Minutes |
|---|---|---|
| 1 | Spinal Rock | 1 |
| 2 | Tree Posture (Vrkasana) | 1 |
| | (*Perform to each side*) | |
| 3 | Back-stretching Posture (Paschimottanasana) | 1 |
| | (*Perform twice*) | |
| 4 | Shoulderstand Posture (Sarvangasana) | 1 |
| 5 | Plough Posture (Halasana) | 1 |
| 6 | (*Perform twice*) Cobra Posture (Bhujangasana) | 1 |

| | | |
|---|---|---:|
| 7 | Cowface Posture (Gomukhasana) | 1 |
| | (*Perform to each side*) | |
| 8 | Relaxation Posture (Savasana) | 2 |
| | Rests and time taken going into and leaving postures | 1 |
| | TOTAL TIME | 10 |

# Abdominal controls in the morning before breakfast

| | **Postures** | **Minutes** |
|---|---|---:|
| 1 | Abdominal Retraction (Uddiyana) | 1½ |
| 2 | Isolation of the Recti (Nauli) | 1½ |
| | Rests and time taken going into and leaving postures | 2 |
| | TOTAL TIME | 5 |

# Sitting postures for a short time daily

Sit cross-legged in Easy Posture (Sukhasana) or Perfect Posture (Siddhasana) or Lotus Posture (Padmasana)

# Advanced postures

As the basic programmes are mastered, other postures may be added to them. Programmes should not exceed thirty minutes. If substituting postures, the following should always be retained because of their great basic value:

### Postures

Spinal Rock
Shoulderstand Posture (Sarvangasana)

Plough Posture (Halasana)
Cobra Posture (Bhujangasana)
Back-stretching Posture (Paschimottanasana) always conclude with
Relaxation Posture (Savasana)

## Breathing exercises

Cleansing Breath (Kapalabhati)
(*two rounds*)
or
Comfortable Pranyama (Sukh Purvak)
(*five rounds*)
Bellows Breath (Bhastrika)
(*three rounds*)
Victorious Breath (Ujjayi)
(*five rounds*)

## Breathing exercises

In warm weather add
Hissing Breath (Sitkari)
(*three rounds*)
Cooling Breath (Sitali)
(*three rounds*)

# _____ Rapid (five minute) _____
# vitalising programme

| Postures | Minutes |
|---|---|
| Yoga Cat Stretch | 2½ |
| Comfortable Pranayama or Cleansing Breath | 2½ |
| TOTAL TIME | 5 |

The Five Minute Programme is for occasional use when time is limited. It is not intended as a permanent substitute for the longer basic programmes.

# 9

# THE ROYAL WAY (RAJA YOGA)

## —————————— Raja Yoga ——————————

Hatha Yoga brings the body into harmony with the universe. The postures and breathing exercises have a calming influence on the mind and prepare it for the disciplines of Raja Yoga – the Royal Path. Hatha Yoga is a preparation for the conquest of consciousness, the mind's turbulence being easiest curbed and its energies concentrated when the body is strong and alert.

Alain Danielou, in a work on the different Yoga ways, says:

'The movements of the mind are the cause of man's bondage. The action of his intellect is the instrument of his freedom. That particular mode of action by which the intellect stills the movements of the mind is known as the Royal Way to reintegration. This is the highest form of Yoga, all other forms being preparatory.'

Romain Rolland has written:

'It (is) astonishing that Western reason has taken so little into account the experimental research of Indian Raja-yogis, and that it has not tried to use the methods of control and mastery, which they offer in broad daylight without any mystery, over the one infinitely fragile and constantly warped instrument that is our only means of discovering what exists.'

## Self-mastery

If you are already carrying out daily Yoga practice you will have experienced its beneficial influence on the mind. The steady, natural postures and smooth, measured Pranayama have a calming and controlling effect on thought and emotion. The meditative exercises of Raja Yoga will complete this mastery.

It takes but a little self-observation to see just how limited is the control over our minds. Raja Yoga teaches mastery of one's mind and self by psychic exercises aimed at controlling and subduing the thought waves or vrittis. The word vritti means literally 'a whirlpool' – and that is just what most people's minds are like.

Harmonious health is impossible if the emotions are not under control. Emotional stresses – worry, fear, frustration, insecurity – are now known to be responsible for such diverse complaints as peptic ulcer, coronary thrombosis, high blood-pressure, tuberculosis, pneumonia, appendicitis, diabetes, asthma and schizophrenia. It has been estimated that in America more than half the people seeking the services of doctors suffer from emotionally induced complaints.

When subjected to stress, the body's glands, in particular the adrenals, release chemicals into the bloodstream which act as resistance mobilisers. When the stress is prolonged, these chemicals turn traitor and can cause serious damage to vital organs. Also bodily resistance to other attacks is lowered.

We can experience for ourselves the harmful and unpleasant effects of such an emotion as anger – the eyes protrude, the face burns, blood pressure rises, the fists clench, the stomach muscles contract. Dark emotions like fear, anxiety, jealousy and hatred poison the bloodstream and destroy health and peace of mind. Medical science now recognises them as killers.

But the bright emotions making for harmony – such as love, joy and hope

– have a beneficial influence on bodily health. The dark emotions contract; the bright emotions expand. Supreme among the latter is love, which if supported by courage will protect you from the stresses of civilisation and lead to a richer and fuller life.

All Yoga practice has the effect of stilling the mind's turbulence and holding the flame of the passions steady. A considerable measure of detachment ('Vairagya' in Yogic terminology) is built up. In Vairagya one does not react automatically to stimuli or impulses, but first relates them to an objective 'I' that decides what the course of action should be. This means that you do not give way to temper or any of the destructive dark emotions. In fact the 'I' kills them before the bodily reaction of flushed skin, tensed muscles and adrenalin-saturated blood has time to take place. Most people are slaves to environmental changes. Even the weather can affect them. The 'I' of ten o'clock is not the 'I' of eleven o'clock; it may not even be the 'I' of one minute past ten, for environmental change of stimuli taking only a split second could trigger off a new mood, a different coloured 'I'. Yoga puts you in touch with your objective 'I' and gives you a permanent centre of gravity. When the world is examined objectively, without heat or passion, one ceases to become so involved with it. Events lose their power to disturb or inflame. Normally it takes much time for old wounds to heal. Such is the miracle of Vairagya that they can heal in a matter of seconds.

All this makes for inner tranquillity. The Yogi may continue to live an active and civilised life, but he will do so calmly and steadily. Sri Aurobindo, in his *Basis of Yoga*, has this to say of the calm mind that results from self-training:

In the calm mind, it is the substance of the mental being that is still, so still that nothing disturbs it. If thoughts or activities come, they do not arise at all out of the mind, but they come from outside and cross the mind as a flight of birds crosses the sky in a windless air. It passes, disturbs nothing, leaving no trace. Even if a thousand images, or the most violent events pass across it, the calm stillness remains as if the very texture of the mind were a substance of eternal and indestructible peace. A mind that has achieved this calmness can begin to act, even intensely and powerfully, but it will keep its fundamental stillness – originating nothing for itself, but receiving from Above and giving a mental form without adding anything of its own, calmly, dispassionately, though with the joy of the Truth and the happy power and light of its passage.

We live in exciting but dangerous times. If we are to come through unscathed we will need the self-mastery that comes from peace of the spirit and having a permanent centre of gravity. The average person does not experience the inner peace and integration of the Yogi. His thoughts are leaves driven hither and thither by the wind of his desires. Through Raja Yoga faithfully practised, the mind can be stilled, thoughts controlled, selected and directed at will. The value of such a mastery in civilised life is obvious.

La Rue puts it: 'Health is wealth; but the very exuberance of bodily health may be a curse without proper mental control. All health that is not ultimately mental is not health at all.'

# East and West

With the last four limbs of Yoga – Pratyahara, Dharana, Dhyana and Samadhi – we leave the external world and enter the internal world of consciousness. This is a natural and easy transition for the Easterner, but many Westerners will stand hesitantly on the brink of what are, to them, uncharted waters. To understand why this is so one must consider the traditional difference between Western and Eastern thought.

Western thought has been directed outwards, concerning itself chiefly with material things. Great advances have been made in such sciences as nuclear physics, but the youngest science and the one in which least progress has been made is that which seeks to understand our own minds – psychology.

The approach of the Eastern thinker, on the other hand, has been philosophical. He has turned his thought inwards, exploring consciousness at the source. While progress to the Westerner means faster travel, more material comforts, and so on, to the Easterner it means spiritual self-revelation. He unhesitatingly leaves the external world to enter the internal world of consciousness, because he feels and believes that the two worlds are one. In entering himself he comes closer to the vast outside universe; external and internal being only relative terms.

'Make peace with yourself,' says St Isaak of Syria, 'and heaven and earth will make peace with you. Endeavour to enter your own inner cell, and you will see the heavens; because the one and the other are one and the same, and when you enter one you see the two.'

As long as we in the West keep turning our attention and energies outwards, there can be no possibility of inner development. The psycho-analyst Dr C. G. Jung has said: 'We have built a monumental world round about us, and have slaved for it with unequalled energy. But it is so imposing only because we have spent upon the outside world all that is imposing in our natures – and what we find when we look within must necessarily be as it is, shabby and insufficient.'

Not only Jung, but many other leading Western psychologists, have studied and appreciated the significance and value of Eastern psychic exploration, among them Professor William James, who said: 'The most venerable system and the one whose results have the most voluminous experimental corroboration, is undoubtedly Yoga. The result claimed, and certainly in many cases accorded by impartial judges, is strength of character, personal power, unshakeability of soul.'

The subconscious is a term beloved of present-day psychologists, writers and journalists. It refers to that part of our minds of which we are not consciously aware, but which nevertheless is the largest part of our minds, and influences to a powerful degree our everyday actions. The subconscious is the storehouse of our memories. Through hypnosis and pyscho-analysis it can be contacted. The ancient Yogis knew about and understood the workings of the subconscious mind thousands of years ago, just as they formulated the philosophic doctrine Syadvada, which resembles relativism, two thousand years before Einstein's discovery.

The idea of meditation, which is the basis of Raja Yoga practice, is strange to the West, unlike the East where not only priests and monks and the very devout set aside time for daily meditation, but also people in all walks of life.

Dr Lily Abegg, in her book *The Mind of East Asia*, says: 'Not only priests and monks take part in the Zen exercises, but also many laymen who wish to study the methods of contemplation. In Japan, particularly during the last war, these attracted large numbers from all sections of the population . . . Not only officers, businessmen and ministers of state, but also postal officials, shop assistants, railwaymen, young schoolboys and many others meditated. It went so far that even in training establishments, school and also in many factories and other concerns a short period was set aside in the mornings for "meditation" (of course not necessarily of a Zen-Buddhist kind!).'

Can you see this happening in the West, where the craze for speed and action leaves no time for so vague and tenuous a thing as meditation? We live lives of hustle and strain, without getting to know our true Self. The Easterner looks on the Westerner as ignorant because he does not know his own nature and is not master of his soul. The Westerner looks on the Easterner as ignorant because he has made little progress in exploring nature and developing the sciences.

Dr Lily Abegg says: 'Our consciousness developed in an extravert, that of the East Asians in an introvert manner. The East Asians followed the inner way and reached a high level of consciousness relatively early; whereas in their knowledge of the world they remained far behind us. They know man better, and we are better acquainted with the world. That is how those mutual accusations of defective knowledge, which are made with complete justification by each side, come about.'

Yet the differences may not be so great as we think. The latest scientific discoveries in the field of nuclear physics, for example, seem merely to corroborate what the ancient East stated in philosophic terms. No race or portion of the globe has the monopoly of wisdom. East can learn from West, and West from East. The outgoing consciousness of the Occident requires the influence of the ingoing consciousness of the Orient. The life-negation of the East requires an awakening from the life-affirmation of the West.

# Levels of consciousness

The aim of Yoga is the attainment of the super-conscious state of samadhi. To this end are the physical preparation of Hatha Yoga and the meditative practices of Raja Yoga devised. The Yogi believes that conscious evolution is inherent in all men. Each one of them possesses the power of spiritual self-unfoldment. Men live in different levels of being, from the animal to the divine. Yoga is the system whereby a man can work in his own lifetime to achieve a higher stage of consciousness.

This idea of different levels of consciousness, though an old one, will be strange to most Westerners. We are inclined to take our consciousness for granted. But is the one we know the only one possible? Does there not seem irrefutable evidence that other people experience different levels of consciousness from ourselves? And have we not had our own moments of heightened consciousness, often in childhood?

Dr Maurice Nicoll says: 'We know that there can enter into all that we see, do, think and feel, a sense of unrealness. Sometimes it takes the form of seeing the unreality of other people. We observe that some force seems to be hurrying everyone to and fro. We see transiently a puppet-world, in which people are moved as by strings. Sometimes, however, in place of unreality, an extraordinary intensity of reality is felt. We suddenly see someone for the first time, whom we have known for years, in a kind of stillness. We perceive the reality of another existence, or we perceive the existence of nature, suddenly, as a marvel, for the first time. The same experience, felt in relation to oneself, is *the sense of one's own existence, independent of everything else,* the realisation of one's indivisibility, the perception of I, of duration without time.

'These feelings surround our natural reality. I think that they show us clearly enough that there are other meanings of oneself, or forms of conscious experience.'

And William James has said: 'Our normal waking consciousness, rational consciousness, is but one special type of consciousness, while all about it, parted from it by the flimsiest of screens, there are potential forms of consciousness entirely different.'

The Gurdjieff/Ouspensky School which has many followers in the West, says that there are seven categories of man.

Man No. 1 is Physical Man. This is an animal man. He identifies his 'I' with his body. The centre of gravity of his psychic life lies in the moving centre. The moving and instinctive functions constantly outweigh the emotional and thinking functions. For him knowledge is based upon imitation or instincts, learned by heart, crammed or drilled into him. He learns like a parrot.

Man No. 2 is Emotional Man. His centre of gravity lies in the emotional centre, the emotional functions outweighing all others. He is the man of feeling, learning by likes and dislikes.

Man No. 3 is Intellectual Man, the man of reason. The centre of gravity of his psychic life is in the intellectual centre, where thinking functions are gaining the upper hand over the moving, instinctive and emotional. His knowledge is that of the book-worm.

All men, says this school, are born one of these three types of men. But by training, self-discipline and strife, higher levels of consciousness can be reached.

Man No. 4 is an intermediate stage. He has become conscious of his possible self-unfoldment. He is beginning to acquire a permanent centre of gravity. One dominant, permanent 'I' is fighting to master the multiplicity of 'I's' that previously struggled for possession of his mind. He is being emancipated from the subjective elements in his knowledge and is beginning to move along the path towards objective knowledge.

Man No. 5 has reached unity. His knowledge is whole, indivisible knowledge. He has one indivisible 'I' and his knowledge belongs to it. What he knows, the whole of him knows.

Man No. 6 differs from Man No. 7 only by the fact that some of his properties have not yet become permanent. Higher centres are at work in him. He possesses powers beyond the understanding of ordinary men.

Man No. 7 has reached the highest stage of conscious evolution. He has free-will and permanent, unchangeable 'I'. He has objective knowledge of ALL.

# Yoga and reason

Raja Yoga, though mystical, is based on the firm foundation of reason. That some schools of Yoga allowed themselves in the course of their long history to become clouded by superstition and magic, does not alter the truth of this basis. Great Yoga teachers like Vivekananda look on Yoga as a science, free from superstition, and based on reason, only in the final stage to transcend it. He says:

To get any reason out of the mass of incongruity we call human life, we have to transcend our reason, but we must do it scientifically, slowly, by regular practice, and we must cast off all superstition. We must take up the study of the super-conscious state just as any other science. On reason we must lay our foundation, we must follow reason as far as it leads; and when reason fails, reason itself will show us the way to the highest plane. When you hear a man say, 'I am inspired,' and then talk irrationally, reject it. Why? Because these three states – instinct, reason and superconsciousness, or the unconscious, conscious, and superconscious states – belong to one and the same mind. There are not three minds in one man, but one state of it develops into the others. Instinct develops into reason, and reason into the transcendental consciousness; therefore not one of the states contradicts the others. Real inspiration never contradicts reason, but fulfils it. Just as you find the great prophets saying, I come not to destroy but to fulfil, so inspiration always comes to fulfil reason, and is in harmony with it.

Raja Yoga does not ask of you anything that is unreasonable. It does not merely theorise, but asks you to try for yourself. Only by putting the technique into practice can you experience its truth.

And if you say that you do not wish to become a mystic, but merely to gain some measure of control over an unruly mind, to enrich that mind and to find tranquillity and strength with which to face an increasingly more complex and difficult life, you will find what you seek in the concentration practices of the Royal Path.

# 10

## — YOGA MEDITATION —

─────────────── **The time** ───────────────

Set aside fifteen to thirty minutes daily for stilling the mind and attaining inner serenity. You will look forward to these periods. The time is not wasted as you will soon discover.

Some students will find two periods of meditation daily highly beneficial. Separate the two meditations by at least six hours.

If you meditate in the morning the inner serenity achieved will be carried into working life. Many readers will object that in the morning they are too rushed. This is often the case but can be overcome by rising earlier so as to fit in the meditation period. This should not be hurried. Give it a trial and you will see how worthwhile it is.

If you meditate before going to bed in the evening the serenity produced will ensure sleep of a high quality. If you go to sleep with worries or active thoughts on your mind you will have poor quality rest, but go to bed with a peaceful mind and you will sleep like a child and awaken wonderfully refreshed in the morning.

Except for two hours after meals, any time of the day will do for Yoga meditation. It is best, once you have decided on a time of day, to stick to it. The habit thus formed assists meditation.

A particularly helpful time to meditate is when called upon to tackle some difficult or fearful task, or when worried or under emotional stress. In the sublime peace of the stilled mind fear and grief and stress are relieved and priceless courage is gained.

# The place

Yoga meditation should be performed in a quiet place free from noise, interruptions and extremes of temperature.

It can be either outdoors or indoors. It is very pleasant to meditate outdoors in peaceful and beautiful surroundings, but weather conditions and other factors may often rule this out.

One place in the house should be decided upon and adhered to. It should be a clean, bright and airy room. It should be without unpleasant associations. Elsewhere, I have told the story of a man who found that he could not relax in a certain room in his house. He felt the presence of some strangely disturbing force. Going over the objects in the room one by one he finally located the trouble. It was a photograph of himself as a child. The trouble was that the photograph showed a little boy with a glorious head of curls, whereas the man was now bald.

Whatever the room you decide upon, you can make its atmosphere more conducive to meditation and relaxation by hanging pleasant paintings on the walls.

# The posture

One of the meditative postures should be used. In these seated poses the body forces are unified and gathered as in a non-leaking container. The work of the lungs and heart is made easier, the body is very still, and the spine – housing the vital nervous system – is held naturally upright.

People who, because of age or any other reason, cannot adopt even the Easy Posture (Sukhasana) should use a comfortable straight-backed chair.

As in performing Pranayama, spine and head should be kept erect and in a straight line. A wall or door may be used for support, and a cushion can be placed against the small of the back to help keep it straight. Sit on a cushion or folded rug or blanket.

If the body and neck muscles are weak the posture will not be firm and steady, both of which are necessary for Yoga meditation. Hence the value of the preparatory Hatha Yoga exercises can be appreciated.

The body must be held perfectly still, naturally braced, yet not tensed. It must not intrude into consciousness. It is a mistake to place oneself in a painfully contorted position and expect to achieve success in stilling the mind. If sense-withdrawal (Pratyahara) is to be achieved there must be no discomfort. This seems obvious, but there are many fanatics who suffer in the difficult Lotus Posture (Padmasana) in the belief that it is the only way to success.

The meditative postures have been proved to be the finest positions for calming and mastering the mind, but remember that the Indian Yogi is familiar with these postures from an early age and spends hours daily thus seated. They are completely comfortable to him. He feels no strain.

If there is any strain at all, make do with the Easy Posture, using a wall or door for back support, or just a chair. Many readers may wonder why lying on your back is not the best position to adopt. It is because a recumbent position would naturally tend to promote a feeling of drowsiness and this is not desirable in Yoga meditation, for in doing it you are not asleep, but rather very much awake and alert.

——— **Curbing the restless mind** ———

In the *Bhagavad Gita* we find the following quotation:

*Arjuna says*: 'For the mind is verily restless, O Krishna; it is impetuous, strong and difficult to bend, I deem it as hard to curb as the wind.'

*Krishna answers*: 'Without doubt, O Mighty-Armed, the mind is hard to curb and restless, but it may be curbed by constant practice and by indifference.'

*Vivekananda says:* 'From our childhood upwards we have been taught only to pay attention to things external, but never to things internal, hence most of us have nearly lost the faculty of observing the internal mechanism. To turn the mind, as it were, inside, stop it from going outside, and then to concentrate all its powers, and throw them upon the mind itself, in order that it may know its own nature, analyse itself – is very hard work. Yet that is the only way to anything which will be a scientific approach to the subject.'

Yes, the mind is difficult to tame, especially if it has been allowed to run loose for many years. But it can be mastered as the *Gita* says 'by constant practice'.

The first step in this practice is Sense-Withdrawal, called Pratyahara by the Yogis.

Remember that Raja Yoga can only be fully understood by living it, by experiencing it for yourself; then what seemed before to be impossibly complex and incomprehensible will be come clear, and progress will be speeded up incredibly.

# —— Sense-withdrawal (Pratyahara) ——

Pratyahara is a detaching of the mind from the sense-organs. The word means 'gathering towards'. It checks the outgoing powers of the mind and turns them inwards. It is a gathering in and integration of the previously scattered mental energies. In Pratyahara one frees oneself from the thraldom of the sense-organs.

When the senses have withdrawn from their objects and transmuted themselves into the modes of consciousness, this is called 'the Withdrawal', Pratyahara (*Yoga Sutras* of Pantanjali 2, 54).

The adept in yoga gives himself up to 'Withdrawal' and stops the traffic of the senses with their objects, which are word, sight, etc., to which they are invariably attached. He then makes his senses work for his Consciousness and the ever-agitated senses are controlled. No yogi can achieve the aim of yoga without controlling the senses. (Vishnu Purana.)

The external world is shut out in Yoga meditation. This detaching from the sense-organs is something that all of us do every day. As I type this sentence, for example, I am conscious only of the idea I wish to express and of the letters tumbling quickly on to the page. Yet now, at the end of it, I can pause and be conscious of so much more. The feel of the chair supporting me, the flickering of the fire whose heat reaches out across the room towards me, birds chirping on the roof-tops outside the house, and so on. To get things done in life we must select our sense impressions, for we are being bombarded by a multiplicity of them every day. We may not be conscious of the ticking of a clock until it stops, then we instantly notice the fact.

The sense-organs themselves are merely the 'middle men' between the external world and consciousness. The eyes, for example, do not see in themselves, but are merely the instrument of consciousness. The real organ of vision is in a nerve centre of the brain. A man may be asleep with his eyes open, yet seeing nothing. Pictures are striking the retinae of his eyes, but the man will not be aware of them because his consciousness is not aroused.

Under hypnosis a person's sense-organs can come completely under the control of the hypnotist. He will tell his subject that his arms feel nothing, and true enough, when a match flame is held to it, nothing is felt. He will tell his subject that a piece of raw potato he is eating is a peach, and the distinct flavour of a peach is experienced. He can open the subject's eyes and make him see whatever he wishes him to see.

Vivekananda, in his *Raja Yoga*, warns against allowing one's mind to become controlled by others. Sense-Withdrawal is something which you must do for yourself, your 'I' must be in complete control. Vivekananda says:

> The faith-healers teach people to deny misery and pain and evil. Their philosophy is rather roundabout; but it is a part of Yoga upon which they have somehow stumbled. Where they succeed in making a person throw off suffering by denying it, they really use a part of Pratyahara, as they make the mind of the person strong

enough to ignore the senses. The hypnotists in a similar manner, by their suggestion, excite in the patient a sort of morbid Pratyahara for the time being. The so-called hypnotic suggestion can only act upon a weak mind. And until the operator, by means of fixed gaze or otherwise, has succeeded in putting the mind of the subject in a sort of passive, morbid condition, his suggestions never work.

Now the control of the centres which is established in a hypnotic patient or the patient of faith-healing, by the operator, for a time is reprehensible because it leads to ultimate ruin. It is not really controlling the brain centres by the power of one's own will, but is, as it were, stunning the patient's mind for a time by sudden blows which another's will delivers to it. It is not checking by means of reins and muscular strength the mad career of a fiery team, but rather by asking another to deliver heavy blows on the heads of the horses, to stun them for a time into gentleness . . .

Every attempt to control which is not voluntary, not with the controller's own mind, is not only disastrous, but it defeats the end. The goal of each soul is freedom and mastery: freedom from the slavery of matter and thought, mastery of external and internal nature. Instead of leading towards that, every will-current from another, in whatever form it comes, either as direct control of organs, or as forcing to control them while under a morbid condition, only rivets one link more to the already existing heavy chain of bondage of past thoughts, past superstitions. Therefore, beware how you allow yourselves to be acted upon by others.

Raja Yoga does not teach morbid introspection or useless daydreaming. There is all the difference in the world between these two states and Pratyahara, Dharana, Dhyana and Samadhi. If a person finds on meditating that he has dozed off or slipped into involuntary reverie, then he should know that he is performing the exercises incorrectly and must bring the wayward attention back to its task. The Raja Yoga mental states are positive and alert.

## —————— Breathing ——————

Pratyahara should be aided by quiet breathing. When we are agitated our breathing is fast and jerky, but if we breathe quietly and evenly tranquillity of mind is promoted. At first you will have to do this deliberately. As you sit motionless in a meditative posture, inhale and exhale slowly through the nose. Let the inhalations and exhalations be long and controlled throughout. This form of breathing during meditation will become a habit; you will no longer be conscious of it, just as you should not be conscious of your seated body.

## — Thought observation and control —

The Yogi seeks to gain control over his thoughts. He seeks the power to select those he considers to be of value and to banish the rest.

People who may be very fussy about what they eat will think nothing of allowing harmful thoughts to dominate their minds.

Mason wrote: 'On the whole, it is of as great importance for a man to take heed what thoughts he entertains, as what company he keeps; for they have the same effect on the mind. Bad thoughts are as infectious as bad company; and good thoughts solace, instruct and entertain the mind, like good company. And this is one great advantage of retirement, that a man may choose what company he pleases from within himself . . . As in the world we oftener light into bad company than good, so in solitude we are oftener troubled with impertinent and unprofitable thoughts, than entertained with agreeable and useful ones: and a man that hath so far lost command of himself, as to lie at the mercy of every foolish or vexing thought, is much in the same situation as a host whose house is open to all comers; whom, though ever so noisy, rude, or troublesome, he cannot get rid of; but with this difference, that the latter hath some recompense for his trouble, the former none at all, but is robbed of his peace and quiet for nothing.'

Resolve now that your mind will no longer be open to all comers, that you will cease to be the slave of your thoughts and desires.

Most of the thoughts that crowd our minds so persistently every day are useless. Each day try and cut down their number. There is no need for excessive will-power to do this, indeed it will only defeat our purpose. As with a wild horse, the mind can only be tamed by gentleness and patience.

Comfortably dressed, in peaceful surroundings, seat yourself in a steady, relaxed posture, and breathe quietly and evenly. Sit perfectly still and try to cut off all sense impressions from without. This is Pratyahara. Wrap yourself as it were in a blanket of silence.

Turn your attention inwards instead of outwards. Allow your thoughts to run through the mind as they please. Now *observe them attentively*. See how they pass in a never-ending stream. See how one thought leads to another, linked by association.

Observe the stream of thought in passive awareness. Feel yourself as a detached 'I' observing your own thoughts just as if they are your fingers or toes or some other parts of the body. As they flow steadily past observe the uselessness of most of them, also their waywardness and lack of unity.

If passive awareness is sustained the thoughts begin to lessen their number. Do not expect a big reduction at once. Do not expect to turn off the mind like an electric light at the touch of a switch. Impatience impedes progress.

You will observe how successive thoughts are linked by association so that they follow immediately upon each other. Separate two thoughts – even for a split second – and you will have a momentary glimpse of the inner stillness that is your goal.

The method of meditation that has just been described – detached observation of the mind – is one of the ways to awareness of the Self beyond the ego.

## ———— The quest for the Self ————

Yoga meditation is designed so that the meditator may uncover his real 'I' or Self. It does not require much self-observation to see that we have a multiplicity of 'I's', each, as Ouspensky says, 'seeking to be Caliph for an hour.' One 'I' makes a New Year resolution, another 'I' breaks it before a week has passed. One 'I' exists at the office, another in the home, a third on the golf course, and so on.

Yet behind all these 'I's' there lies the central 'I', pure consciousness, an objective centre of gravity from which our body, our emotions, and our very thoughts themselves can be observed. Man, as far as we know, is the only living thing capable of this level of consciousness. The body, the feelings, the intellect itself, can be set aside as 'not I' things.

'Pursue the enquiry "Who am I?" relentlessly,' advised an Indian guru, Sri Ramana Maharashi. 'Analyse your entire personality. Try to find out where the I-thought begins. Go on with your meditations. Keep turning your attention within. One day the wheel of thought will slow down and an intuition will mysteriously arise. Follow that intuition, let your thinking stop and it will eventually lead you to the goal.'

We have already seen that, both involuntarily by hypnosis and voluntarily by Pratyahara, the sense-organs can be cut-off from their centres of consciousness. A burning match applied to the back of the hand of a hypnotised person may not be felt. Some Yogis detach themselves to such an extent from their bodies that they can be buried alive, drink poison, or walk through fire, without coming to any harm. Such exhibitionistic fanaticism is deplored by genuine Yogis, but it does show the extent to which the body ceases to count with a person who is firmly established in the Self. Such a person does not feel cold or heat, pain or pleasure.

Similarly we can learn to detach ourselves from the negative emotions such as anger, envy, jealousy and unjustified fear. In man's early quest for survival these emotions served a life-preserving purpose, but in present-day civilised life they are in the main repressed and harmful to health and peace of mind. Anger, for example, floods the bloodstream with chemicals which mobilise the body for fight. But, except in war, one can no longer expect to destroy one's enemies physically. Anger also brushes aside reason and makes us act in ways that we may later regret. Efficient living is impossible without emotional control, and Yoga promotes just such a mastery.

Just as we can observe both body and emotions as 'not I' things, so the thought-observation exercises described earlier in this chapter will enable you to experience the intellect as an instrument of the Self, and the instrument of your conscious evolution.

The non-Self is the body, senses and mind. That which perceives the non-Self is the real Self.

> The Purusha, no bigger than a thumb, is the inner Self, ever seated in the heart of man. He is known by the mind, which controls knowledge, and is perceived in the heart. They who know Him become immortal . . .

> His hands and feet are everywhere; His eyes, heads, and faces are everywhere; His ears are everywhere; He exists compassing all.

> Himself devoid of senses, He shines through the functions of the senses. He is the capable ruler of all; He is the refuge of all; He is great . . .

> The Self, smaller than the small, greater than the great, is hidden in the hearts of creatures. The wise, by the grace of the creator, behold the Lord, majestic and desireless, and become free from grief.

> (*Svetasvatara Upanishad*, III, 13, 16, 17, 20.)

And in knowing the Self (Atman) the Yogi knows the universal Overself (Brahman).

That thou are (tat twam asi).

# 11

# YOGA — CONCENTRATION — AND CONTEMPLATION

'To maintain the mind fixed on one spot is called concentration' (*Yoga Sutras* of Patanjali, 3, 1).

When by Pratyahara the tyranny of the sense has been checked, it becomes easier for the mind's energies to be focused on one point. This action, in Yoga, is called Dharana. Raja Yoga develops this power of concentration to an intense degree which can lead to psychic powers, though these powers are not its aim.

The power of the mind is greatest when instead of its forces being scattered they are brought together and focused on a point. This bringing to bear of the full weight of the intellect on a subject can result in intuitive knowledge or revelation. The Yogis say that many of the great Western inventors and intellectual giants of the past hit on Raja Yoga methods by accident or actually practised them not knowing that they did so.

Dharana is another step on the path to Self-realisation. Yoga writers have compared the mind to the surface of a pool, which is constantly troubled and in motion because of the agitation of our thoughts. If we can still this flow of thoughts and hold the mind steady, then pure consciousness, our inner Self, will be revealed and seen at the bottom of the pool. Patanjali says that Yoga is restraining the mind-stuff (Chitta) from taking various forms (Vrittis). The Chitta can be compared to the surface waters of a pool, and the Vrittis are the thought waves that cross it.

# ———— Aid to successful living ————

The ability to concentrate sharply to bring all your attention to the task in hand or the object of study, is one of the greatest keys to successful living. The man with highly developed powers of concentration can get through a tremendous amount of work. He can work with great efficiency. He can study with great intensity.

The great artist is lost in his work. All his attention is directed towards the canvas. All his faculties are brought to bear on the task in hand.

Concentration is one of the chief secrets of success in games and on the sports field. Watch the star footballer about to take a penalty kick, the master golfer attempting a long putt, the skilled snooker player about to pot a critical black. All three will have one thing in common . . . intense concentration!

'Genius is concentration,' said Schiller.

The concentrative energies of the mind will be aided if in daily life you give your full attention to things. Most people go through life in a sort of waking-sleep. The Yogi gives his full attention to even the smallest task, and at the same time manages to be very alive and alert. This is termed, in Yoga, Samprajanya or Awareness.

# ———— Concentration exercises ————

The Yogi stills the mind and makes it steady by focusing it to a point just as the rays of the sun are captured and brought to a point of burning intensity by means of a magnifying glass. To achieve this feat various aids may be employed.

One of these is to focus your gaze on some object. It is best if the object is small rather than large.

If you are meditating outdoors you may choose a flower, a bush on a distant hill, a small, white cloud suspended motionless in a sky of amethyst, a stone protruding from the swirling waters of a mountain stream.

If you are indoors you may choose an ornament, a flower in a vase, an apple, perhaps a brightly shining star observed in the evening from a bedroom window. You may choose a photograph of a pleasant scene or of a loved one, or a painting of a religious subject or landscape of great beauty. You can make your own choice and try several until you find those that most appeal to you. Patanjali says in one of his Sutras that the Yogi can meditate on 'anything that appeals to one as good'.

Whatever object you choose it is best to focus the gaze on some central point. The attention should be directed to this spot as a torch-beam illuminates one spot in a dark room and is rested there steadily yet impalpably. If you use a portrait photograph, gaze into the eyes of the person. If you use a landscape painting, fix your gaze on a tree or some other object.

At first you will be sure to find that you cannot keep your attention on the object for very long. The mind will wander off into involuntary reverie. Suddenly, perhaps minutes later, you will 'wake up' from your reveries to realise that the object of concentration has been entirely neglected. You stare at the object for a while but soon it is forgotten. You are thinking instead about what you will do tomorrow, what happened that afternoon, the show you saw last night, your job, income tax, the state of the world . . . anything but the object of concentration. Don't get angry with yourself. Don't become tensed up about it. Instead, gently coax your attention back to its task. Great force is not required in this work. Considerable effort will tire you and defeat your purpose. It is a fault if the face is screwed up and the body muscles are tensed in concentration.

Let us see an example of Yoga concentration at work, taking for our object something simple and pleasant – an apple. The technique followed here has been found by the author to give the best results.

Set the apple eighteen inches (46 cm) before you on the ground, or on a low stool or table. Let it be a handsome apple with a smooth, well-polished skin. If you can have a light shining on it so much the better.

Now examine the apple with all your senses. Do this slowly, thoroughly.

Study the apple's appearance: its size, shape, texture and colouring. See how when you study it closely you find that it has not just one or two colours as you thought at first, but numerous colours. There is yellow there, and green and brown and russet and red. There is a dent where it has fallen, ripened by the sun, on the lush orchard grass. Now lift it to your face and feel its cool, smooth skin against your cheek. Touch it lightly with your lips. Smell its clean, fresh tang.

Then set it down again before you, keeping your gaze focused steadily upon it. Now start thinking about it: how it grew, how it ripened in the sun, how it dropped from the tree, how it was packed and despatched to the wholesaler who sold it to the shop where you bought it.

No superfluous thoughts must be allowed to intrude into this concentrated examination of the apple. If they do, push them gently aside and bring the attention back to its task.

# Dhyana

Having exhausted all possible thoughts about the apple, the next stage is no longer to think about the size, shape, texture, colouring, smell, feel or history of the apple, but to fix in the mind the single idea *apple*, the essence distilled as it were from the previous few minutes' thought. With the eyes still fixed steadily on the apple, hold the idea *apple* unwaveringly in the mind. This is Dharana proper. Hold it for some time and you will attain the next Yoga limb, Dhyana, which if maintained for several minutes can lead to Samadhi, when the perceiver and the thing perceived have become one.

When the mind's energies are focused on a selected point and held there, so that but one thought wave, steady and straight, disturbs the surface of the mind-stuff (Chitta), this is called Contemplation (Dhyana). When Contemplation is maintained for some time, even this one remaining wave fades away and the untroubled, superconscious state of Samadhi ensues.

# Visualisation

Up to now we have been dealing with Dharana practised with the eyes open so as to fix the gaze on some object; later you should concentrate with the eyes closed. This banishes external sense-impressions, making Pratyahara and the one-pointing of the mind easier. The object should then be held before the mind's eye.

Most people can with a little practice acquire the necessary powers of visualisation. We each possess within us a private mental cinema on whose screens we project our hopes, fears and memories. Without having to travel to a well-loved beauty spot, and without spending a single penny, a person with strongly developed powers of visualisation is able to transport himself to that place and see it clearly before his inner eye. He can see it in detail and in colour, and if his imagination is lively he will hear the sounds appropriate to the scene, the singing of birds or the sound of the wind or the sea.

The development of such powers of visualisation is well worthwhile, apart from its use in Raja Yoga. It means you can store up a private collection of pictures which can be enjoyed at any time. Scenes of great beauty which you witnessed on your holidays, the look on the face of a child or a loved one . . . all these need not be lost in the maw of devouring time, but captured and filed away in your mental projection room for the rest of your life.

Still using an apple for our example as the object of concentration, the meditator may study it intently for a while, then close his eyes and still picture the apple, clearly showing behind the closed lids. After some practice at this the actual apple may be dispensed with and only its inner reflection used. The same applies to any other objects you may use for Dharana.

Many Yogis fix their inner gaze on the space between the eyebrows, or some other part of the body.

In the *Bhagavad-Gita* we find:

> Shutting out the external contact with the sense-objects, the eyes fixed between the eyebrows, and equalising the currents of Prana (incoming breath) and Apana (the outgoing breath) inside the

nostrils, the meditative man, having mastered the senses, mind and intellect, being freed from desire, fear and anger, and regarding freedom as his supreme goal, is liberated forever.

In Dharana, consciousness can be directed to any part of the body. If you think of a spot on the palm of your hand and concentrate intensely on it for some time, it will begin to redden and burn just as if the rays of the sun were being focused there by a magnifying glass. The powers of the mind are developed to such an extent by adepts that even the sympathetic nervous system comes under the control of the will. They can control the beating of the heart, for example. This has been authentically proved many times. The advanced Yogi is able to direct his consciousness to any part of his body, external or internal, and hold it there.

# Auto-control using biofeedback equipment

Recently, in the West, experiments using electrical biofeedback equipment have shown that ordinary men and women can duplicate, with only a few hours of training, some of the feats of the Yogis in controlling physiological processes normally controlled by the involuntary nervous system. The heart rate can be slowed down, the blood pressure can be lowered and brain wave rhythms can be altered to order. Subjects are trained to produced Alpha waves and the patterns of brain activity found in EEG (electro-encephalograph) studies of meditating Yogis, Zen monks, and Transcendental Meditators. The mind in the Alpha state is neither active nor drowsy, but in the 'middle tone' known to meditators. Most subjects find the Alpha rhythms soothing.

We must be careful not to assume that because some physiological changes associated with Yogic meditation can be duplicated, then the auto-control of biofeedback monitoring and the state of consciousness of meditation are the same. Nevertheless, the use of biofeedback methods offers a fascinating field for investigation. Two American psychologists have written that 'the ultimate possibilities of a man's self-control are nothing less than the evolution of an entirely new culture where people can change their mental and physiological states as easily as switching channels on a television set.'

## The mystic sounds

Sounds may be used to hold the attention in Yoga meditation. You may concentrate on the ticking of a watch in a quiet room; or, if outdoors, you may close your eyes and listen to the sound of a waterfall or a purling stream. Old Yoga texts speak of the air being charged with cosmic energy (prana) in the vicinity of lakes and rivers. In fact, we know today that the air in such regions is heavily charged with negative air ions which impart a feeling of vitality to consciousness.

Some gurus instruct their pupils in the art of concentrating on inner sounds (nadas). The ears are closed with the fingers and the attention is focused on the sounds that are heard. With practice the mind is able to hold on to progessively finer and subtler sounds, until eventually liberation is achieved.

Here are the *Hatha Yoga Pradipika*'s instructions on listening to the nadas or mystic sounds.

The sound which a muni (sage) hears by closing his ears with his fingers should be heard attentively, till the mind becomes steady in it. By practising with this nada, all other external sounds are stopped. The Yogi becomes happy by overcoming all distractions within fifteen days. In the beginning, the sounds heard are of a great variety and very loud; but as the practice increases, they become more and more subtle. In the first stage, the sounds are surging, thundering like the beating of kettledrums, and jingling ones. In the intermediate stage, they are like those produced by conch, Mridanga, bells, and so on. In the last stage, the sounds resemble those of tinklets, the flute, Vina, bees, and so on. These various kinds of sounds are heard as being produced in the body. Though hearing loud sounds like those of thunder and kettledrums, etc., one should try to get in touch with subtler sounds only. Leaving the loudest, taking up the subtle one, and leaving the subtle one, taking up the loudest, thus practising, the distracted mind does not wander elsewhere.

Wherever the mind attaches itself first, it becomes steady there; and then it becomes absorbed in it. Just as a bee, drinking sweet juice, does not care for the smell of the flower; so the mind, absorbed in the nada, does not desire the object of enjoyment. The mind, like an elephant, habituated to wander in the garden of enjoyments, is capable of being controlled by the sharp goad of anahata nada (heart sound). The mind, captivated in the snare of nada, gives up all its activity; and, like a bird with clipped wings, becomes calm at once. Those desirous of the kingdom of Yoga, should take up the practice of hearing the anahata nada, with mind collected and free from all cares.

## ———— Contemplation of the void ————

This is described by the *Siva Samhita* as a practice sure to bring Self-realisation.

Let him (the Yogi) contemplate on his own reflection in the sky as beyond the Cosmic Egg: in the manner previously described. Through that let him think on the Great Void unceasingly. The Great Void, whose beginning is void, whose middle is void, whose end is void, has brilliancy of tens of millions of suns, and the coolness of tens of millions of moons. By contemplating continually on this, one obtains success. Let him practise with energy daily this dhyana, within a year he shall obtain all success undoubtedly. He whose mind is absorbed in that place even for a second, is certainly a Yogi, and a good devotee, and is revered in all worlds. All his stores of sins are at once verily destroyed. By seeing it one never returns to the path of this mortal universe; let the Yogi, therefore, practise this with great care by the path of Svadhishthana. I cannot describe the grandeur of this contemplation. He who practises, knows.

# — Contemplation of the inner light —

Patanjali gives as one of the things to be meditated upon, 'The Effulgent Light'.

In Samadhi a great white light may be seen, the colourless light of pure consciousness. Sitting in a meditative posture, perfectly still, with eyes closed and senses withdrawn, the Yogi may concentrate until perceiving a small point of light before the mind's eye. By concentrating the mind's energies on it, it will grow until he becomes filled with it and Super-consciousness occurs.

# A Tibetan technique

Some Yogis use a meditative technique in which the mental image of a flower, tree or person is held for a time, then gradually demolished, bit by bit, until only a clear light remains. This technique is described in *The Tibetan Book of the Dead*, edited by Evans-Wentz.

> Whosoever thy tutelary deity may be, meditate upon the form for much time – as being apparent, yet non-existent in reality, like a form produced by a magician . . . Then let the vision of the tutelary deity melt away from the extremities, until nothing at all remaineth visible of it; and put thyself in the state of the Clearness and the Voidness – which thou canst not conceive as something – and abide in that state for a little while. Again meditate upon the tutelary diety; again meditate upon the Clear Light; do this alternately. Afterwards allow thine own intellect to melt away gradually, beginning from the extremities.

# Blotting out the Ego

A similar technique requires the meditator to feel his closed eyes and his head to be filled with foaming water. Next he must meditate on his body from the throat to the stomach, filling it with imaginary water. Then he mentally fills all of his body, including the arms and legs, with cool water, the colour of glass. After he has filled all of himself with pure water, he should imagine that the room too is filled with it. When this has been clearly experienced, he must gradually drain away the water, reversing the previous process. That is to say, he drains the water from the room slowly and steadily until none remains between ceiling and floor; then from his arms, legs and stomach; next from his chest and throat; finally from his head and eyes. In this way the false Ego vanishes.

# A world of diamonds

In yet another method to achieve withdrawal and onepointedness, the meditator imagines that he has a diamond in each ear, and a canopy of diamonds about his head, and that all his surroundings, whether outdoors or indoors, have been turned into diamonds (or crystal), bright, pure, clean and shutting out all sound.

# Japa

In Mantra Yoga the mind is concentrated by means of Japa, the repetition of sacred syllables, words and prayers (mantras). The Japa may be voiced (vachika), whispered (upanshu), or mental (manasa), the last being considered the highest.

The sacred syllable OM (AUM) is considered the finest mantra. The Upanishads describe it as being a symbol of the whole universe and 'all that is past, present and future . . . and whatever else there is, beyond the threefold division of time.'

'Meditate on Atman as AUM'; 'AUM, this word, is Brahman.'

# ———— Taittirya upanishad ————

AUM is considered to be the basis of all sound – the 'a' is formed far back in the throat, the 'u' carries the tone forward, and the word leaves the mouth from the closed vibrating lips. Its vibrations are said to be beneficial to health and the disciplining of the mind.

Other mantras frequently used are Soham (He is I), and Hansah (I am He).

# ——— Transcendental Meditation ———

Transcendental Meditation – TM, as it is known for short – is a streamlined form of mental (manasa) repetition of a mantra. The method was brought to the West by Maharishi Mahesh Yogi in 1959, and the tiny, chuckling guru became a household name in America and Europe during temporary associations with stars of the entertainment industry. The method is simple. You sit comfortably and mentally repeat a Sanskrit word provided by a TM instructor on initiation. Each time the attention wanders from the word, calmly bring it back. The effortlessness of the meditation is stressed. Progress may be checked with the instructor. A fee is charged for initiation.

The claim to special skills in selecting a secret personal word for each meditator – in fact, many meditators may use the same mantra – does not appear to be borne out by the study of Dr Herbert Benson at the Harvard Medical School. Dr Benson says: 'Tests at the Thorndyke Memorial Laboratory of Harvard have shown that a similar technique used with any sound or phrase or prayer or mantra *brings forth the same physiologic* changes noted during Transcendental Meditation.' However, the *Maharishi* follows an age-old tradition in the East that certain sounds produce specific effects. And the physiological effects are only one aspect of meditation.

Transcendental Meditation has been devised to suit busy Westerners and it has proved effective in inducing deep bodily and mental relaxation.

# 12
# PSYCHIC POWERS (SIDDHIS)

## — Samyama —

The last three limbs of Yoga – concentration, meditation, and absorption – when practised together with regard to one object, are called Samyama. An object is selected and dwelt upon; the stage of concentration relaxes into effortless meditation, which leads to absorption and unitary consciousness. Professor Ernest Wood, in his *Yoga* (Penguin Books), translates Samyama admirably as 'mind-poise,' and says: 'Such an idea is not to be confused with checking, still less with check-mating or stoppage. It does, however, involve a unified poise with reference to the object or idea at a given time under review or treatment. It involves, as poise always does, whether in poetry or in the dance, an elimination of irrelevancies. Poise is dynamic – something quite different from pose, which is static.' The dynamic character of making Samyama on an object or idea goes a long way to explaining Yoga's reiterated claim to engendering psychic powers (Siddhis).

What happens in Samyana has resemblances to deep contemplations upon a landscape, a flower, a painting, or selections of prose or poetry that are profoundly meaningful. The landscape, the flower, the painting, or words are gone over in their parts, then all the parts are 'brought together' (one definition of Samyama), and finally the whole is contemplated, a whole greater than the sum of its parts.

In advanced practice, the Yoga meditator progresses from mind-poise on concrete objects to mental processes and finally to the Self or Atman, opening up mystical consciousness.

Though the reality of psychic powers is spoken of quite often by the Yoga masters, they warn against giving them too much attention and importance, whereby they could become obstacles to progress on the Royal Way. Patanjali himself, though giving quite a lot of space to them in view of the conciseness of his *Sutras*, warns: 'These are obstacles to Samadhi; but they are powers in the worldly state.' (111,38.) The possession of Siddhis could so easily intensify the ego and harden it, whereas the Yogin seeks to transcend it. Similar warnings against 'special powers' are given by Zen masters, Sufi masters, Christian mystics, and so on. The common instruction of the mystic teachers is that psychic powers should be looked upon as wayside objects on the spiritual journey and should not be allowed to become ends in themselves.

## ——— Extra Sensory Perception ———

The old Yoga texts frequently mention such psychic faculties as telepathy, clairvoyance and premonition. In the third part of his *Yoga Sutras*, Patanjali lists thirty-seven psychic powers resulting from the application of the 'inner limbs' of concentration, meditation and absorption. 'Making Samyana on' various body parts, ideas and qualities is said to produce occult powers – 'to become small as an atom', 'going through the skies', 'to have one's desires fulfilled', and so on – which some commentators take literally and others symbolically. On the claim that the practice of Yoga meditation favours the triggering of powers of extra sensory perception (ESP), much support can be found in modern scientific research.

Recent research studies have shown that the relaxed meditative state of mind is conducive to the display of ESP. It is significant that the best results arise in subjects who have relaxed body and mind, let go and opened up to a state of passive receptivity. Some researchers believe that we all – or nearly all – have psychic abilities that are normally overwhelmed by activity ('noise') in the nervous system; calm the nervous system and the latent powers may awaken. This view is supported by experiments in sensory deprivation. In what are known as *Ganzfeld* experiments, sound and touch stimuli are reduced to a minimum and the eyes receive uniform 'white light'. (A *Ganzfeld* is a uniform, homogeneous visual field.) These conditions have been found to favour success in ESP tests.

Interestingly, in Yoga meditation – and other Eastern forms of meditation – the approach is also through sense-withdrawal (Pratyahara) and quietening of activity in the nervous system, producing a mental state that is frequently likened to the reflecting surface of a mirror or lake. And EEG (electroencephalograph) readings of the electrical brain activity of subjects in successful ESP experiments have shown the slow Alpha waves also associated with states of deep relaxation and meditation.

# Kundalini Yoga

This esoteric Yoga – also called Laya (Latent) Yoga – aims at awakening powerful psychic energies and developing psychic powers that are linked with activating energy centres belonging to the subtle or astral body. Such training needs a qualified instructor. By concentrating on seven main centres, or chakras (literally 'wheels'), situated between the base of the spine and the brain, one can attain superconsciousness by arousing what is symbolically termed 'the coiled serpent' Kundalini, said to be asleep in the first or root centre at the base of the spine. It is described by some writers as electricity, a negative pole being freed and racing up to unite with the positive pole in the brain. This power, when aroused, can be passed up the centre of the spine, from chakra to chakra, until it reaches the top of the head, when superconsciousness is achieved. Great psychic powers are said to result from this Yoga, but readers should be warned that it could be dangerous unless practised with guidance from a highly qualified Yoga master.

The Kundalini passes upwards through a channel situated in the centre of the spine and called the Sushumna-Nadi. Two other Nadi run alongside it, the negative Ida-Nadi on its left and the positive Pingala-Nadi on its right. Investigators state that the Yoga chakras are approximate with centres of bunched nerve ganglia in the body; others approximate the chakras with the chief bodily glands. Such explanations are inadequate, and it is more satisfactory to view Kundalini as an occult Yoga and the Nadi, chakras and so on as belonging to the subtle or astral body.

The Yogis have named each centre, and the awakening of Kundalini is assisted by visualising the chakras as coloured lotus flowers, each with seed-syllables and other symbols.

## The Chakras

1  **The Root Centre** (Muladhara)
   Situated just above the anus, at the very base of the spine. It is here that the coiled energy lies sleeping.
2  **The Support of the Life Breath Centre** (Svadishthana)
   Situated in the genital area.
3  **The Jewel City Centre** (Manipura)
   Situated in the region of the navel.
4  **The Unstruck Sound Centre** (Anahata)
   Situated in the heart.
5  **The Great Purity Centre** (Vishuddha)
   Situated in the throat.
6  **The Command Centre** (Ajna)
   Situated in the middle of the brow.
7  **The Thousand Petalled Lotus Centre** (Sahasrara)
   At the crown of the skull. The Centre of Self-realisation.

There are several secondary chakras: Lalana, situated between the Vishuddha and Ajna Centres; Brahmarandhra, situated just above the Ajna Centre; Manas, close to the Ajna Centre; Soma, just above the Manas chakra; Karanarupa, a group of 'seven casual forms' situated near the Ajna Centre; and Manipitha, situated above the 'seven casual forms'.

# 13

# SELF-
# —— REALISATION ——
# (SAMADHI)

We come now to Samadhi, the last of Patanjali's eight limbs of Yoga.

Directing attention upon one place is concentration (Dharana), the sixth of limb of Yoga.

Attention flowing evenly and effortlessly in one direction is contemplation or meditation (Dhyana), the seventh limb of Yoga.

When consciousness becomes one with the object being contemplated, so that there is no awareness of the ego-self, that pure state of existence is Self-realisation (Samadhi). Other translations for Samadhi are Identification, Absorption, and Realisation.

Though it is not true of all meditators, many experienced meditators learn to recognise certain signs preceding the onset of Samadhi. There is a feeling of very deep relaxation without sensation of body or mind. This 'off-sensation' is known by meditators of many cultures. Katsuki Sekida, a Zen Buddhist, writes: 'It is not a state of numbness, for you can move your limbs and body if you want. But if you keep your body still, it is not felt. This condition I call "off-sensation". In this state the activity of the cortex of the brain becomes steadily less and less, and we can regard this condition as a Preliminary to entering Samadhi . . . Subsequently, by stilling the activity of our mind, a state is reached in which time, space, and causation, which constitute the framework of consciousness, drop away. We call this condition "body and mind fallen off". In ordinary mental activity the cerebral cortex takes the major role, but in this state, apparently, it is hardly active at all. "Body and mind fallen off" may seem to be nothing but a condition of mere being, but this mere being is accompanied by a remarkable mental power, which we may characterise as a condition of extreme wakefulness.' (*Zen Training*, Weatherhill, New York and Tokyo.) The term Samadhi for the state of pure consciousness is used by the Buddhists as well as by the Hindus. Trance states of probably an auto-hypnotic character, as in Yogis who allow themselves to be buried alive for many hours, are sometimes called Samadhi – but the peak of Yogi meditation is of a different nature and characterised by clarity and wakefulness. There is simple pure existence. Words and thoughts and images are absent. Time and space are transcended. Body and mind are quiescent and filled with peace. This state has the clarity of white light and great purity – 'light' is the metaphor most frequently used by men and women who have experienced Samadhi at its purest.

## The Self

The Self or Self-realisation is not the ego-self but the Atman of Indian philosophy. To know the Self beyond the ego is to uncover Being. The experience is described as Sat (Being) – Chit (Consciousness) – Ananda (Bliss). Ramana Maharshi, who answered thousands of questions put to him by people seeking enlightenment, said that though these three aspects of Realisation go together, a person's approach to Self-realisation led to emphasis on one of the three. In the combined Hatha Yoga/Raja Yoga approach of this book, the experience of consciousness (Chit) will be strongest. Samadhi is a fourth state of consciousness, higher than that of sleep without dreaming, sleep with dreaming or ordinary waking consciousness.

Replying to a questioner who asked about Samadhi, Ramana Maharshi described it as 'remaining in the primal, pure, natural state without effort' and added that 'the only permanent thing is Reality, and that is the Self.' He also called the Self the 'I-am'. 'That is the abiding and fundamental Reality. This truth was taught by God to Moses. "I *am* that I-am".'

Ramana Maharshi also said: 'Once attained, the state of Self-realisation is the same by whatever path and whatever religion it may be approached.' (*The Teachings of Ramana Maharshi,* Rider.).

Two important stages of Samadhi are described as 'with seed' and 'without seed'. The second stage comes when even the idea of control is absent, having faded away. If we think of our mind as a pool and of thoughts as the waves that cross its surface, then Dharana reduces all waves to a single one; Dhyana maintains it fixed for some minutes at a stretch, and with Samadhi 'with seed' the wave is reduced to the gentle one that is the thought of control itself. When even this wave fades away, advanced Samadhi has been achieved.

Vivekananda explains it:

You remember that our goal is to perceive the Soul Itself. We cannot perceive the Soul because It has got mingled up with nature, with the mind, with the body. The ignorant man thinks his body is the Soul. The learned man thinks his mind is the Soul; but both of them are mistaken. What makes the Soul get mingled up with all this? Different waves in the Chitta rise and cover the Soul; we only see a little reflection of the Soul through these waves. So, if the wave is one of anger, we see the Soul as angry; 'I am angry,' one says. If it is one of love, we see ourselves reflected in that wave, and say we are loving. If that wave is one of weakness, and the Soul is reflected in it, we think we are weak. These various ideas come from these impressions, these Samskaras covering the Soul. The real nature of the Soul is not perceived as long as there is one single wave in the lake of the Chitta; this real nature will never be perceived until all the waves have subsided; so, first, Patanjali teaches us the meaning of these waves; secondly, the best way to repress them; and thirdly, how to make one wave so strong as to suppress all other waves, fire eating fire as it were. When only one remains, it will be easy to suppress that also; and when that is gone, this Samadhi or concentration is called seedless. It leaves nothing, and the Soul is manifested just as It is, in Its own glory.

Later (in *Raja Yoga*) he says:

. . . in this first state of Samadhi (Samadhi with seed) the modifications of the mind have been controlled, but not perfectly, because if they were, there would be no modifications. If there is a modification which impels the mind to rush out through the senses, and the Yogi tries to control it, that very control itself will be a modification. One wave will be checked by another wave, so it will not be real Samadhi, in which all the waves subside, as control itself will be a wave. Yet this lower Samadhi is very much nearer to the higher Samadhi than when the mind comes bubbling out.

This same distinction is found in Zen-Buddhist meditation, where you have the two stages of 'present-heart' (Ushin) and 'no-heart' (Mushin), heart here meaning consciousness.

The Zen-Buddhist, Daisetz Suzuki says:

If you are possessed by certain thoughts, then your heart is to that extent closed to other thoughts. If you are occupied, then you can neither hear nor see anything, but if you keep your heart empty, that is to say open, then you can take in everything which approaches you – that is what is called Mushin. If, however, you are only concerned with keeping your heart empty, this very condition of your heart will prevent you from realising Mushin or the original heart. Herein lies the difficulty of attaining the state of no-heart. But when your practising reaches maturity it comes about of its own accord. You cannot hasten this state of Mushin. As an old poem has it: 'Being mindful of not-thinking is thinking nevertheless. O that I were now beyond thinking and non-thinking.'

## Samadhi: Its nature

To the Yogi the Postures (Asanas), Breathing Exercises (Pranayama), Sense-withdrawal (Pratyahara), Concentration (Dharana), and Contemplation (Dhyana) are but steps in a journey up a mountainside. Raja Yoga provided the final moves to the pinnacle of supreme bliss . . . Samadhi.

What is this Samadhi so earnestly sought?

It is given many names: Union, Integration, Identification, Liberation, Superconsciousness, Realisation, Self-realisation. It is an inner peace in whose radiance one can bask. It is above and beyond the senses. Words, therefore, cannot adequately describe it. It must be experienced.

At the point where Samadhi is reached the Ego ceases to exist. All sense of 'I' and 'mine-ness' is banished. It is a liberation from the tyranny of desires, fears, worries, persons, places and things.

Note this description of Ramakrishna attaining the culminating stage of Nirvikalpa Samadhi:

> The Universe was extinguished. Space itself was no more. At first the shadows of ideas floated in the obscure depths of the mind. Monotonously a feeble consciousness of the Ego went on ticking. Then that stopped too. Nothing remained but existence. The soul was lost in Self. Dualism was blotted out. Finite and infinite space were as one. Beyond word, beyond thought, he attained Brahman.

You will appreciate this better if you think of those moments in your life when you experienced the most sublime happiness. Am I not right in thinking that they were those moments when the Ego was annihilated, when you were 'carried out of yourself' by an emotional experience, the sight of a glorious sunset or landscape, the sound of glorious music, a moment of truth?

The poet Tennyson spoke of: 'A kind of waking trance I have frequently had, quite up from boyhood, when I have been all alone. This has generally come upon me through repeating my own name two or three times to myself, silently, till all at once, as it were, out of the intensity of consciousness of individuality, the individuality itself seemed to fade away into boundless being, and this not a confused state, but the clearest of the clearest, the surest of the surest, utterly beyond words, where death was almost a laughable impossibility, the loss of personality (if so it were) seeming no extinction but the only true life . . . I am ashamed of my feeble description. Have I not said that the state is beyond words?'

Those readers who have cultivated a love of beautiful things will understand what is meant. Poets, artists and musicians have been touched at times by the divine breath. And we too may have experienced it in those moments – very often in childhood – when we are carried out of ourselves on being confronted by the beautiful and the wonderful. Visvanatha has said: 'The experience of beauty is pure, self-manifest, compounded equally of joy and consciousness, free from admixture of any other perception, the very twin brother of mystical experience, and the very life of it is supersensuous wonder.'

'All art,' wrote Walter Paters, in *The Renaissance*, 'constantly aspires towards the condition of music.'

Perhaps in the language of music the voice of Superconsciousness can be heard. J. W. N. Sullivan stated that great composers like Beethoven were able in their music 'to communicate valuable spiritual states which testify to the depth of the artist's nature and to the quality of his experience of life.' (*Beethoven*, Alfred A. Knopf, New York).

Music can elevate the spirit and blot out the Ego. Observe an audience held spell-bound by great music. Note how still they are, how relaxed, how steady their gaze on conductor, singer or performer.

Music lovers will know that there is often experienced a sudden upsurge of elation at certain moments in their favourite works.

One of my favourite records is 'Death of a Novice' (La Mort De L'Escola), sung unaccompanied in Catalan by the Orfeo Catala de Barcelona.

In this record the voice range from the purest boy-soprano to the most profound and deepest of bassos. These latter imitate the tolling of the funeral bell.

There is a point near the end of the work when the voices are suddenly quiet. There is a pause, a silence, then a boy-soprano commences to sing in a voice of pure silver, a shaft of radiant light that suddenly stabs into the semi-darkness of the cathedral.

At that moment I always experience a rapid outgoing of fear, desire, worry and egoism, with a resultant relaxation and inrush of ineffable peace. There is Samadhi – perhaps only for a second – but a second of such richness as to be beyond time or measurement.

Earlier, unrevised versions of this book contained the above account of my personal response to a favourite record, without further comment. The result was that people wrote from many parts of the world pointing out that the record had been deleted from the manufacturer's catalogues and pleading, in tones of desperation, for me to send them tape recordings of the music. I had not thought it necessary to explain that I was describing a personal response to a recording that altered consciousness *for me* and that I was not recommending the record as a key to instant Samadhi *for all*. I should add now that with frequent hearings the record would not have had the effect described. I now listen to it at intervals of several months and only when an inner sense tells me that it is a propitious time to do so. Even then the effect is not always as rewarding as occurred in my earliest hearings.

There are other moments in listening to favourite music that often have a similar ego-transcending effect for me, but readers must find the moments in music that are transcendental for themselves, giving glimpses of pure existence. They may occur in listening to so-called classical music, to jazz, to a folk song or to popular music in some form.

With Samadhi we enter a region of pure being where attempts at description in the rational terms of language must necessarily be inadequate. We have the evidence of those who have experienced it most profoundly that it is 'beyond words'. Nevertheless, C. F. Morel makes a praiseworthy attempt at an explanation in rational terms: 'Consciousness is . . . something intensely mobile. When the exterior world has disappeared, the circle of consciousness contracts and seems to withdraw entirely into some unknown and usually ignored cortical centre. Consciousness seems to gather itself together, to confine itself within some unknown psychic pineal gland and to withdraw into a kind of centre wherein all organic functions and all psychic forces meet, and there it enjoys unity.' And Theos Bernard assures us that it 'is not an imaginary or mythical state, though it is explained by myths, but is an actual condition that can be subjectively experienced and objectively observed.'

Mouni Sadhu, in his *In Days of Great Peace* (Allen and Unwin Ltd.), says that Samadhi has three phases:

'*The First* – when we feel it is approaching. In this state we can still move and talk as usual. We can compare it to early twilight before sunrise.

'*The Second* can be compared to the midday when the sun stands high in the sky. Then the mental and physical functions decline, they become dreamy, and *reality* alone, independent of all form and condition, dawns upon and illumines our being. We then *know Who we are*, we are above and beyond them. We breathe freedom, bliss and wisdom.

'*The Third* – which comes immediately after our "coming back" from

Samadhi – is like the second twilight, this time preceding sunset. We still feel in ourselves its last rays, we still clearly remember the *light*, but its vivid reality gradually fades away when we return to our "normal" consciousness, the waking state. But the remembrance of Samadhi is not completely lost. We are still unable to stay in its permanently, due to our imperfect spiritual development, but henceforth we *know* irrefutably that this state exists, that it *is* in truth, the only reality. After experiencing Samadhi even once we are different beings.'

Those who have achieved mystical enlightenment are agreed on several things: Samadhi is a positive and not a negative state like sleep or hypnotic trance; and it is distinguished by two features – an altered conception of time, and the experiencing on a level of being of the unity of all life.

# ———— Living in the now ————

When the mind is stilled by Raja Yoga, time – that is to say, *psychological* time – ceases to exist. For time is relative: it only exists when one thing is taken in relation to another. If I go on a train journey my leaving the train at my destination, taken in relation to my getting in, shows a passage of time. Similarly, if I think of 'fruit', and in a split second follow with another thought 'apples', then time has passed, and I am aware of its passing. But if the mind takes one thought and holds it, one-pointed and still, time is erased, it ceases – psychologically – to exist.

In the hurly-burly of civilised living we rarely find time, or even give a thought to living in the *NOW*. We spend our *NOW* in thinking of the past or dreaming of the future. Raja Yoga enables us to be still and experience eternity, as defined by Boethius: 'to hold and possess the whole fullness of life in one moment, here and now, past and present and to come.'

'No reveries, no conversations, no tracing out of the meaning of fantasies, contain this *NOW*, which belongs to a higher order of consciousness,' writes Dr Maurice Nicoll, in his *Living Time and the Integration of the Life*. 'The *time-man* in us does not know *NOW*. He is always preparing something in the future, or busy with what happened in the past. He is always wondering what to do, what to say, what to wear, or what to eat. He anticipates; and we, following him, come to the expected moment, and lo, he is already elsewhere, planning further ahead. This is *BECOMING* – where nothing ever *IS*. We must come to our senses to begin to feel *NOW*. We can only feel *NOW* by checking this time-man, who thinks of existence in his own way. *NOW* enters us with a sense of something greater than passing time. *NOW* contains all time, all the life, and the aeon of the life. *NOW* is the sense of higher space. It is not the decisions of the man in time that count here, for they do not spring from *NOW*. All decisions that belong to the life in time, to success, to business, comfort, are about 'tomorrow'. All decisions about the right thing to do, about how to act, are about tomorrow. It is only what is done in *NOW* that counts, and this is a decision always about *ONESELF* and *WITH* oneself, even although its effect may touch other people's lives 'tomorrow'. *NOW* is spiritual. It is a state of the spirit, when it is above the stream of time-associations. Spiritual values have nothing to do with time. They are not in time, and their growth is not a matter of time. To retain the impression of their truth we must fight with time, with every notion that they belong to time, and that the passage of days will increase them. For then it will be easy for us to think it is *TOO LATE*, to make the favourite excuse of passing time.

'The feeling of *NOW* is the feeling of certaintly. In *NOW* passing time halts, and in this halting of time one's understanding has power over one. One knows, sees, feels in oneself, apart from all outer things; and above all, one *IS* . . . All insight, all revelation, all illumination, all love, all that is genuine, all that is real, lies in *NOW* – and in the attempt to create *NOW* we approach the inner precincts, the holiest part of life. For in time all things are seeking completion, but in *NOW* all things are complete.'

## Unity

To the Yogi Samadhi is the merging of the individual Soul or Self with the universal Soul or Overself.

In the *Siva Samhita* we find:

As space pervades a jar both in and out, similarly within and beyond this ever-changing universe there exists one Universal Spirit.

Having renounced all false desires and chains, the sannyasi and Yogi see certainly in their own spirit the Universal Spirit.

Having seen the spirit that brings forth happiness in their own spirit, they forget this universe, and enjoy the ineffable bliss of Samadhi.

The meaning of the saying 'That thou art' (Tat twan asi) is realised on reading this dialogue from the *Chandogya Upanishad*:

'When Svetaketu was twelve years old he was sent to a teacher, with whom he studied until he was twenty-four. After learning all the Vedas, he returned home full of conceit in the belief that he was consummately well educated, and very censorious.

His father said to him, "Svetaketu, my child, you who are so full of your learning, and so censorious, have you asked of that knowledge by which we hear the unhearable, by which we perceive what cannot be perceived, and know what cannot be known?"

'"What is that knowledge, sir?" asked Svetaketu.

'His father replied, "As by knowing one lump of clay all that is made of clay is known, the difference being only in name, but the truth being that all is clay – so, my child, is that knowledge, knowing which we know all."

'"But surely these venerable teachers of mine are ignorant of this knowledge; for if they possessed it they would have imparted it to me. Do you, sir, therefore give me that knowledge."

'"So be it," said the father . . . And he said, "Bring me a fruit of the nyagrodha tree."

'"Here is one, sir."

'"Break it."

'"It is broken, sir."

'"What do you see there?"

'"Some seeds, sir, exceedingly small."

'"Break one of these."

'"It is broken, sir."

'"What do you see there?"

'"Nothing at all."

'The father said, "My son, that subtle essence which you do not perceive there – in that very essence stands the being of the huge nyagrodha tree. In that which is the subtle essence all that exists has its self. That is the True, that is the Self, and thou, Svetaketu, art That."

'"Pray, sir," said the son, "tell me more."

'"Be it so, my child," the father replied; and he said, "Place this salt in water, and come to me tomorrow morning."

'The son did as he was told.

'Next morning, the father said, "Bring me the salt which you put in the water."

'The son looked for it, but could not find it; for the salt, of course, had dissolved.

'The father said, "Taste some of the water from the surface of the vessel. How is it?"

'"Salty."

'"Taste some from the middle. How is it?"

'"Salty."

'"Taste some from the bottom. How is it?"

'"Salty."

'The father said, "Throw the water away and then come back to me again."

'The son did so; but the salt was not lost, for the salt exists forever.

'Then the father said, "Here likewise in this body of yours, my son, you do not perceive the True; but there in fact it is. In that which is the subtle essence, all that exists has its self. That is the True, that is the Self, and *thou*, Svetaketu, *are That*."'

Unity, completeness, wholeness, integration – this is the goal of all esoteric teaching; and those who work to attain the highest levels of consciousness can experience the universe as the unity its name implies.

Western science is coming more and more to provide evidence of a physical basis for the intuitive knowledge of the Eastern mystic.

'Separate, individual existences are illusions of common sense,' says Aldous Huxley, in *Ends and Means*. 'Scientific investigation reveals – and these findings, as we shall see later on, are confirmed by the direct intuition of the trained mystic and contemplative – that concrete reality consists of the inter-dependent parts of a totality and that independent existences are merely abstractions from that reality.' And later: 'More recently investigators, trained in the discipline of mathematical physics and equipped with instruments of precision, have made observations from which it could be inferred that all the apparently independent existences in the world are built up of a limited number of patterns of identical units of energy. An ultimate physical identity underlines the apparent physical diversity of the world. Moreover, all apparently independent existences are in fact interdependent. Meanwhile the mystics had shown that investigators, trained in the discipline of recollection and meditation, could obtain direct experience of a spiritual unity underlying the apparent diversity of independent consciousness. They made it clear that what seemed to be the ultimate fact of personality was in reality not an ultimate fact, and that it was possible for individuals to transcend the limitations of personality and to merge their private consciousness into a greater, impersonal consciousness underlying the personal mind.'

What Huxley says is borne out by the interesting report of the Peckham biologists: ' . . . plant, animal and man live by the same biological law. The laws that govern growth and development apply equally to the organism as a whole, or to its parts . . . the process of diversification so characteristic of organism and, as a result of the life process, equally apparent in the environment, must denote some PROGRESSIVE ORDER in the latter. Can it be that the environment, also *in process*, is taking on an orientation as ordered as that which the embryologist can follow so clearly in the differentiation of the embryo – like the chick developing from the amorphous material of the egg? Is, then, the process we call "evolution", with all its manifest expressions, but one universal expression of the *organisation* of the environment itself? Is the environment ALIVE?

'The mutual action of organism and environment, associated as we rise in the biological scale with an increasing degree of autonomy of the organism, recalls forcibly to mind the circumstances of a single cell, such as for instance the liver-cell, set in the body of which it is an infinitesimal part. The cell acts as liver cell carrying on the specific function of *liverness*, yet always, in health, *aware* of, and subject to, the wider needs of the body of which it is part and from which it derives sustenance. It is the RELATIONSHIP TO THE BODY which alone gives significance to its individuality as liver cell as well as to its unique function of liverness.

'The pathologist is only too familiar with the situation that arises where this delicately poised relationship of the cell's autonomy within the sphere of a greater organisation – the body – is absent. When the cell multiplies without reference to the impulses of the greater organisation of the body of its inhabitation, the result is cancer, the definition of which might be stated as "multiplication without function" – loss of individuality. Such procedure ushers in antagonism, disrupting the mutual association between the cell and its environment – and ends in the ultimate destruction of the cell, of the body in which it grows, or of both.

'Thus the body as an organisation is, in fact, the ultimate significance of the cell. Can it then be that Man himself is but a cell in the body of Cosmos; and that Cosmos is organismal as he is?

'Without being able to define the factual basis of their intuition – for that can only come through science – wise men in all ages have acted with a deep intuitive consciousness of this as truth. Upon it they have built their hopes, their conduct and their religions. Only now, as intuitive apprehension seems to be wearing thin and threadbare, are men of science being led, through the study of function, to suspect that there may even be a physical basis for these primitive intuitive actions; that in fact the significance of human living lies in the degree of MUTUALITY established with an all pervading order, Nature – whether we deify her or not.'

Here we have Western scientists reporting that indeed man may bc – as the Eastern Yogi says – microcosm in macrocosm.

# 14

# – AFTER REALISATION –

Patanjali's eight limbs of Yoga, which provided a useful structure for this book, may mislead in one respect. It is easy to think of the limbs as rungs of a ladder or steps up the side of a mountain or a pyramid. You keep morally pure; you sit with symmetrical stability in a meditative posture and you perfect your body by posture, breathing exercises, personal hygiene and diet; you control breathing and prepare the mind for meditation and while meditating you breathe gently, evenly and rhythmically; you cut down on the distractions of sense stimuli by turning the attention inwards and settling into yourself; you gather your powers of attention and rest them upon a single object or idea, which provides a constant stimulus; you keep the attention on target until awareness is effortless and smooth; and finally meditation flows into pure existence (Samadhi). From one point of view it is helpful to see these as successive stages; but the analogy with rungs and steps does not satisfactorily meet the total picture. Self-realisation contains all the preceding limbs, and one returns from it into ordinary consciousness, descending the ladder, as it were. And during meditation, if I might be permitted to change metaphors, awareness may dive deep into the ocean bed several times and between times return at least part way to the surface. There is a further consideration: how much of the Samadhi state 'sticks', suffusing ordinary consciousness? A wheel or a circle might make a better image than that of steps.

YOGA

Maharishi Mahesh Yogi, in an Appendix to his translation of Chapters one
to six of the *Bhagavad Gita* (Penguin Books), in which he puts forward
many challenging interpretations of the text, says of Patanjali's eight
limbs of Yoga that each relates to a sphere of life. 'With the continuous
practice of all these limbs, or means, simultaneously, the state of Yoga
grows simultaneously in all the eight spheres of life, eventually to
become permanent.'

Whether the Maharishi gives the right interpretation or not, it is agreed
by persons in the best position to know, because of their experience in
such states, that repeated dips into pure consciousness lead to an
infusion of its qualities into every moment and activity of living. This
would indeed produce changes in the functionings connected with the
other limbs. Yoga masters exemplify such changes: their normal life
reflects non-violence, contentment, and the other qualities Patanjali
refers to in the first two limbs; their posture is marked by poise and
naturalness (Zen monks have been known to attain sudden enlightenment on seeing a Zen Master eat rice or put on his sandals); their
breathing is quiet, smooth, and rhythmical; they cope easily with sense
stimuli; they effortlessly sustain concentration (the whole person wholly
attending), which passes into contemplation and on into serene Samadhi.
Their everyday actions are marked by poise and tranquillity.

We have referred to Self-realisation as the goal of Yoga – but it is also a
beginning. Leaving that state of pure being we return to living in the
relative fields of everyday activity. For some time the experience of
Realisation may fade following meditation – but if the experience is
repeated regularly it may eventually become permanent and be present
in every action. Maharishi Mahesh Yogi uses an apt analogy on this
matter. He likens the dips into pure being, experienced during meditation, to dipping cloth in vegetable dye; at first the colour fades in the sun;
but with repeated dippings the colour stays fast. Similarly, there is a
stage beyond Samadhi, which the Maharishi and mystics of various
cultures call Cosmic Consciousness. This permanent state is spoken and
written of in Zen and in other traditions of meditation. In it every moment
partakes of the quality of pure being experienced in meditation.

Ramana Maharshi told a questioner: 'When, through practice, we are
always in that state, in going into Samadhi and coming out again, that is
the Sahaja state. In Sahaja one sees the only Self and sees the world as a

form assumed by the Self . . . In this state you remain calm and composed during activity. You realise that you are moved by the deeper real Self within and are unaffected by what you do or say or think. You have no worries, anxieties or cares, for you realise that there is nothing that belongs to you as ego and that everything is being done by something with which you are in conscious union.'

The state of permanent consciousness attained by the Realised Man that Ramana Maharshi spoke of is a far-off goal for most practitioners of Yoga. However, Yoga practice produces more rapid changes, many of which have already been described in the course of this book. Many readers should already have had their first taste of them.

Some of the changes that result in persons using Yoga methods are obvious to their friends. They look, and are, healthier, brighter of eye and clearer of skin. They are more composed, relaxed, courteous, tactful, humble, and tolerant. Their self-mastery earns the respect of others. They are clearly more at peace with themselves and with the universe of which they are a part.

Hatha Yoga prepares the body and the mind for the spiritual exercises of Raja Yoga. No other system so perfectly and effectively realises the ideal of *mens sana in corpore sano*, a sound mind in a sound body. Yoga shows the way to physical and mental well-being. It integrates. It promotes a balanced personality. It puts the whole being into harmony with the universe. (Health, it should be noted, may be defined as 'wholeness'.)

With the feeling of unity that Yoga practice establishes comes an awakening of reverence for life and of love towards all living things.

In conclusion, it should be said that, as with other practices, results are proportionate to the amount of effort expended.

As the *Hatha Yoga Pradipika* says:

'Whether young, old or too old, sick or lean, one who discards laziness gets success if he practises Yoga. Success comes to him who is engaged in the practice; for by merely reading books on Yoga, one can never get success. Success cannot be attained by adopting a particular dress. It cannot be gained by telling tales. Practice alone is the means of success.'

# GLOSSARY

**Ahimsa**   Non-violence
**Ajna**   Command Chakra
**Akasha**   Ether
**Anahata**   Unstruck Sound Chakra
**Apana**   Outgoing breath
**Agarigrapha**   Non-possessiveness
**Ardha-Matsyendrasana**   Twist Posture
**Ardha-Sarvangasana**   Half-Shoulderstand Posture
**Ardha-Sirsasana**   Half-Headstand Posture
**Asanas**   Postures
**Asteya**   Non-stealing
**Atman**   The individual spirit; the Self

**Basti**   Colonic Irrigation; one of the six purification practices
**Bhakti Yoga.**   Union by devotion
**Bhastrika**   Bellows Breath
**Bhujangasana**   Cobra Posture
**Brahman**   The Overself; the Supreme Reality; the universal spirit

**Chakra**   Centre of psychic energy; literally 'wheel'
**Chakrasana**   Wheel Posture
**Chitta**   Mind stuff

**Dhanurasana**   Bow Posture
**Dharana**   Concentration
**Dhauti**   Stomach cleansing; one of the six purification practices
**Dhyana**   Contemplation

**Gomukhasana**   Cowface Posture
**Guru**   Yoga master

**Halasana**   Plough Posture
**Hansah**   I am He
**Hatha Yoga**   Union by bodily control

**Ida**   Left nostril
**Ishvara Pranidhana**   Attention to the Divine

**Jalandhara**   Chin-lock
**Janusirasana**   Knee and Head Posture
**Japa**   Repetition of sacred syllables, words and mantras
**Jnana Yoga**   Union by knowledge

**Kaivalya**   Isolation
**Kapalabhati**   Cleansing Breath
**Kumbhaka**   Breath suspension
**Kundalini**   Latent energy; 'the coiled serpent'

**Manipura**   Jewel City Chakra
**Mantra Yoga**   Union by sound
**Mantras**   Prayers
**Matsyasana**   Fish Posture
**Mayurasana**   Peacock Posture
**Muladhara**   Root Chakra
**Muni**   Sage

**Nadas**   Mystic sounds
**Nadis**   Nerve channels of the subtle body
**Nauli**   Isolation of the recti muscles
**Neti**   Nasal cleansing; one of the six purification practices
**Nirlamba Sarvangasana**   Balancing Shoulderstand Posture
**Niyamas**   Observances

**Om (Aum)**   Sacred syllable; symbol of Atman and Brahman; the
basis of all sound

**Padhahasthasana**   Standing Forward Bend Posture
**Padmas**   Lotus Posture
**Parbatasana**   Mountain Posture
**Paschimottanasana**   Back-stretching Posture
**Patanjali**   'The father of Yoga'; author of the Yoga Sutras
**Pingala**   Right nostril
**Prana**   The life force; incoming breath
**Pranayama**   Breath control
**Pratyahara**   Sense withdrawal
**Puraka**   Inhalation
**Purusha**   The inner self

**Sahasara**   Thousand Petalled Lotus Chakra
**Salabhasana**   Locust Posture
**Samadhi**   Self-realisation; Absorption; Identification; Super-consciousness; the highest stage of Yoga practice
**Samprajanya**   Awareness
**Samyama**   The last three limbs of Yoga practised together: concentration, contemplation, absorption
**Santosha**   Contentment
**Sarvangasana**   Shoulderstand Posture
**Satya**   Truthfulness
**Shat Karma**   The Purification Practices
**Siddhus**   Adepts
**Siddhasana**   Perfect Posture
**Siddhis**   Supra-natural powers
**Simhasana**   Lion Posture
**Sirsasana**   Inverted Body Posture; Yoga Head Stand
**Sitali**   Cooling Breath
**Sitkari**   Hissing Sound Breath
**Soham**   He is I
**Sukhasana**   Easy Posture
**Sukh Purvak**   Comfortable Pranayama
**Sunya**   The void
**Supta-Vajrasana**   Pelvic Posture
**Svadhishthana**   Support of Life Breath Chakra
**Svadhyaya**   Study
**Syadvada**   Philosophic doctrine resembling relativism

**Tapas**   Austerity

**Trataka**   Eye cleansing; one of the six purification practices
**Trikonasana**   Triangle Posture

**Uddiyana**   Retraction of the abdominal muscles
**Ujjayi**   Audible Breath

**Vajrasana**   Thunderbolt Posture
**Vairagya**   Detachment
**Vishuddha**   Great Purity Chakra
**Vrittis**   Thought waves
**Vrksasana**   Tree Posture

**Yoga**   Union; 'to yoke'; merging of the Self with universal Overself
**Yogasana**   Yoga Posture
**Yogin**   Male Yogi (alternative term)
**Yogini**   Female Yogi (alternative term)

# SELECT BIBLIOGRAPHY

Aurobindo, Sri, *Basis of Yoga*, Sri Aurobindo Ashram, PONDICHERRY, 1936.

Behanan, Kovoor T., *Yoga: A Scientific Evaluation*, Macmillan, reissued Dover Publications, NEW YORK, 1937.

Benson, M. D., Herbert, *The Relaxation Response*, William Morrow, NEW YORK, 1976.

Bernard, Theos, *Hatha Yoga: Heaven Lies Within*, Rider, LONDON, 1950.

Brahmachari, Dhirendra, *Yogasana Vijnana*, Asia Publishing House, LONDON, 1970.

Danielou, Alain, *Yoga: the Method of Re-Integration*, Christopher Johnson, LONDON; University Books, NEW YORK – both 1949.

Edgerton, Franklin, *The Bhagavad Gita*, Oxford University Press, LONDON, 1944.

Evans-Wentz, W. Y., ed. *The Tibetan Book of the Dead*, Oxford University Press, LONDON, 1927.

Hewitt, James, *The Complete Relaxation Book* and *The Complete Yoga Book*, Rider, LONDON, 1982 and 1983; *Teach Yourself Meditation* and *Teach Yourself Relaxation*, Hodder and Stoughton, LONDON, 1978 and 1985.

Huxley, Aldous, *The Perennial Philosophy*, Chatto and Windus, LONDON, 1946.

Iyengar, B. K. S., *Light on Yoga*, Allen and Unwin, LONDON, 1966.

James, William, *Varieties of Religious Experience*, Longmans, LONDON, 1902.

Karlins, Marvin and Lewis M. Andrews, *Biofeedback: Turning on the Power of Your Mind*, Garnstone Press, LONDON, 1973.

Kingsland, Kevin and Venika, *Hathapradipika*, Grael Communications, NEW YORK, 1971.

Lysebeth, Andre Van, *Yoga Self Taught*, Harper, NEW YORK; Allen and Unwin, LONDON, both 1971.

Mahesh Yogi, Maharishi, *On the Bhagavad Gita*, Penguin Books, LONDON, 1969; *The Science of Being and Art of Living*, SRM Publications, LONDON, 1963.

Mascaro, Juan, trans. *The Upanishads*, Penguin Books, LONDON, 1965.

Muller, Max, trans. *The Upanishads*, Clarendon Press, OXFORD, 1898.

Nicoll, Maurice, *Living Time and the Integration of the Life*, Vincent Stuart, LONDON, 1952.

Patanjali, trans. Manilal Nabhubbai Dvivedi, *Yoga Sutras*, MADRAS, 1890.

Pearse, Dr Innes H. and Crocker, Lucy H., *The Peckham Experiment*, Allen and Unwin, LONDON, 1943.

Phelan, Nancy and Michael Volin, *Yoga For Women*, Stanley Paul, LONDON, 1963.

Radhakrishnan, S., *The Bhagavad Gita*, Allen and Unwin, LONDON, 1948; *The Principal Upanishads*, also Allen and Unwin.

Ramana Maharshi, ed. Arthur Osborne, *The Teachings of Ramana Maharshi*, Rider, LONDON, 1962.

Rele, V. G., *The Mysterious Kundalini; Yogic Asanas*, D. B. Taraporevala, BOMBAY, 1927.

Rieker, Hans-Ulrich, trans. *The Yoga of Light; Hatha Yoga Pradipika, India's Classical Handbook*, Allen and Unwin, LONDON, 1972.

Sadhu, Mouni, *In Days of Great Peace*, Allen and Unwin, LONDON.

Sekida, Katsuki, *Zen Training*, John Weatherhill, NEW YORK, 1975.

Sen, K. M., *Hinduism*, Penguin Books, LONDON, 1961.

Sinh, Pancham, trans. *Hatha Yoga Pradipika*, Lalit Mohan Basu, The Panini Office, ALLAHABAD, 1915.

Sullivan, J. W. N., *Beethoven: His Spiritual Development*, Alfred A. Knopf, NEW YORK, 1927.

Taimini, I. K., *The Science of Yoga*, Theosophical Publishing House, Wheaton, ILLINOIS, 1967.

Vasu, Sris Chandra, trans. *Gheranda Samhita*, Adar, MADRAS, 1933.

Vidyarnava, R. B. S. Chandra, trans. *Siva Samhita*, Sudhindra Nath Basu, The Panini Office, ALLAHABAD, 1923.

Vivekananda, Swami, *Raja Yoga, or Conquering the Internal Nature*, Advaita Ashrama, CALCUTTA, 1901.

Wood, Ernest, *Yoga*, Penguin Books, LONDON, 1959.

# INDEX

# MEDITATION

## JAMES HEWITT

Meditation helps you to maintain physical health and mental clarity with equanimity. It is the key technique in the search for higher consciousness and, as such, plays a vital role in many of the world's religions and the pursuit of psycho-physical relaxation.

James Hewitt provides a clear, concise and practical guide to meditation as practised in both East and West. He is not solely concerned with one tradition or school, but explores the different methods of meditation and encourages you to experiment to find the one that suits you best.

**TEACH YOURSELF**

# RELAXATION

## JAMES HEWITT

This book explains the benefits of natural relaxation and provides a practical guide to techniques for enhancing mental and bodily self-awareness – the key to neuromuscular relaxation and control.

The author presents two simple, daily programmes for reducing tension and coping calmly with the pressures of life. Separate chapters are devoted to rapid relaxation techniques, body posture and poise, promoting natural sleep and coping with emotional stress. Alternative techniques – including meditation, biofeedback, hypnosis and autogenic training – are also described. Throughout, the emphasis is on finding the techniques which work best for you in reducing anxiety and stress and promoting a healthier, more relaxed lifestyle.

**TEACH YOURSELF**

# ZEN
## a way of life

## CHRISTMAS HUMPHREYS

This well-known introduction to Zen explains and points the way to the experience of Zen, bringing heightened consciousness, spiritual fulfilment and enlightenment.

With this book, Christmas Humphreys, founder of the Buddhist Society, London – now the oldest and largest Buddhist organisation in Europe – has made an important contribution to the understanding of Zen. He begins by discussing the basic doctrine of Buddhism and the expanded principles of Mahayana Buddhism. Having described the background to the Zen school of Buddhism, he turns to Zen itself and examines the actual process of self-training towards the Zen experience of Reality.

## TEACH YOURSELF